D0251648

The
G.I. Handbook

The
G.I. Handbook

Glycemic Index
How the glycemic index works

Barbara Ravage

BARRON'S

First edition for the United States,
its territories and possessions, and Canada
published in 2005 by
Barron's Educational Series, Inc.
by arrangement with
The Ivy Press Limited

Copyright © THE IVY PRESS LIMITED, 2005

All rights reserved. No part of this book may be reproduced in any form,
by photostat, microfilm, xerography, or any other means, or incorporated
into any information retrieval system, electronic or mechanical, without
the written permission of the copyright owner.

Disclaimer
The views expressed in the book do not necessarily reflect those of the
author of the Foreword, or of The Dr. Robert C. Atkins Foundation.

All inquiries should be addressed to:
BARRON'S EDUCATIONAL SERIES, INC.,
250 Wireless Boulevard
Hauppauge, New York 11788
www.barronseduc.com

ISBN-13: 978-0-7641-3160-8
ISBN-10: 0-7641-3160-5

Library of Congress Catalog Card No. 2004113058

This book was conceived,
designed, and produced by
THE IVY PRESS LIMITED
The Old Candlemakers
West Street, Lewes
East Sussex, BN7 2NZ, U.K.

Creative Director   *Peter Bridgewater*
Publisher   *Sophie Collins*
Editorial Director   *Jason Hook*
Design Manager   *Simon Goggin*
Designers   *Fineline Studios*
Illustrator   *John Woodcock*
Picture Researcher   *Joanna Clinch*
Project Editor   *Mandy Greenfield*

Printed in China
9 8 7 6 5 4 3 2

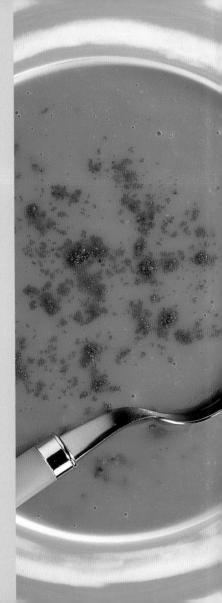

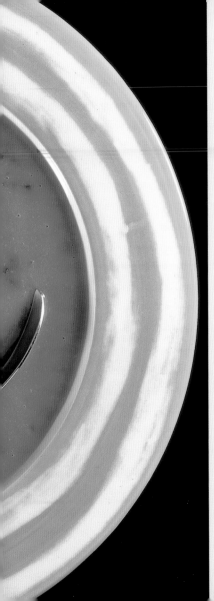

Contents

Foreword

For decades I and many other nutrition/dietetic practitioners and health professionals have attempted to create enthusiasm about good dietary habits, proper food choices, and healthy eating. It wasn't until very recently, however, that the topic gained popular attention and polarized both the medical establishment and the public. Many clinicians, Dr. Robert Atkins most prominently, and researchers such as Dr. David Jenkins, who is also an out-of-the-box thinker, practice, publish, and strongly advocate the need for dietary change and a shift in focus from the low-fat dogma that took hold of the nation at large and seemed to develop a life of its own to a change in carbohydrate consumption.

The basic concept that carbohydrates in our diet have an impact on our health, our weight status, and our nutritional levels has been established and supported by a large body of literature. This has led to evolving debates within the scientific community about the nature of carbohydrates: the effect of low-glycemic vs. high-glycemic foods; how many grams of dietary (ingested) carbohydrates are needed for obligatory regulation of organs and cells; or what percent of carbohydrate is needed for optimal health, adequate nutritional intake, or energy needs.

As the scientific community began to recognize the need to address the questions being posed about carbohydrate and its effects on the metabolic function and physiologic impact of the body, studies to address these issues were undertaken. As a result, evidence-based findings that support clinical experiences have begun to emerge. Numerous studies evaluating the impact of foods with varying glycemic effects on blood glucose and insulin levels have shown differences in the metabolic responses to varying foods with different glycemic indices.

It must be noted that despite the emerging research, a large segment of the medical community still does not accept the concept of differentiating food choices based on glycemic index or load. The topic is still evolving. Similarly, the question of whether one derives benefit from decreasing total grams of carbohydrate or decreasing only the choice of carbohydrate foods to maintain a low glycemic impact on blood glucose and insulin levels has not been fully embraced by the nutrition community to date. However, several studies are in progress that may soon shed light on this specific issue.

Healthy eating is not, of course, just about clinical studies. The underlying mechanisms and responses by the body to food are very complicated and complex. Laboratory measures and clinical trials affect the responses compared to those of real-world experiences. Foods are not eaten in isolated circumstances. Food combinations are not typically considered when one sits down to a meal or grabs a snack. Therefore, studying the impact of foods and meals on one's body can be very challenging and frustrating. What *The G.I. Handbook* offers is a simple system of assessing the glycemic index of different foods to enable you to study and adapt your approach to a healthy diet as an alternative, an option to the current prevailing recommendation.

It is clear that our dietary practices and approaches over the past several decades have failed us. Therefore, it might be time to push the envelope, test the suggestions offered in the following pages, and then observe the outcome. You might be very surprised at the results.

Abby S. Bloch, PhD, RD
Nutrition Consultant, NYC
Vice President, Programs and Research
The Dr. Robert C. Atkins Foundation

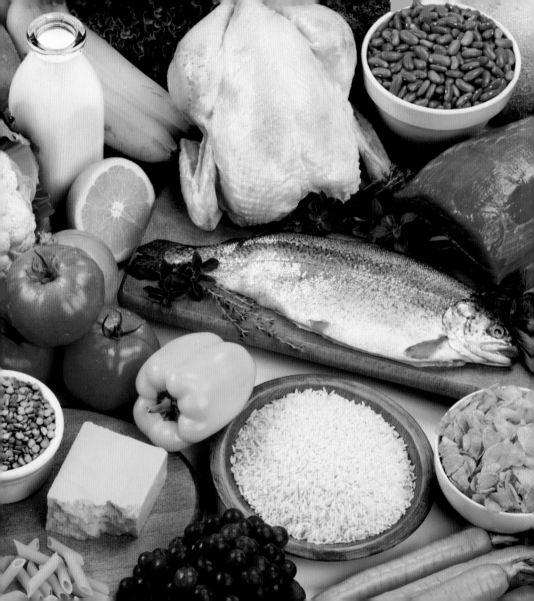

Introduction

We've all heard the latest news: carbohydrates are the enemy. Avoid them like the plague. But *are* carbs really bad? *Is* it safe to eat all fat all the time? *Is* pasta passé? What about fiber and antioxidants, beta-carotene and phytochemicals, and all the other healthy nutrients found most abundantly in grains, fruits, and vegetables—the very carbohydrate foods that have gotten such a bad rap? What is a health-conscious consumer to do?

An Essential Tool

The answer is *The G.I. Handbook*, a compact guide that will help you navigate the murky waters of the latest diet fads. It makes sense of the whole carbohydrate controversy, no matter which diet you are following or what your goals are.

The glycemic index—G.I. for short—is not a diet. It is a tool for healthy eating. And it is a tool that works whether you want to lose weight or maintain a hard-won weight loss; fuel a morning run or support a weight training program; control your blood sugar or reduce your risk of life-shortening illnesses such as heart disease, diabetes, high blood pressure, and even some cancers. It works for women and men who want to get in shape, and for parents who want their children to avoid the poor eating habits that lead to a lifetime of obesity and ill health. It can be particularly valuable for teens, whose bodies are changing and whose nutritional requirements demand more than snack food and fast food can provide.

A wide world of wonderful food awaits you when the G.I. guides your eating choices.

So Many Diets

Bookstores, newsstands, and the Internet are awash with new diet strategies. These days, the overwhelming majority of them are based on controlling carbohydrate intake to one degree or another. Most distinguish between "good" carbs and "bad" carbs, and a whole new language has sprung up, featuring such "nutri-speak" terms as *net carbs*, *carb impact*, and *white carbs*. The focus has changed from cutting fat and counting calories to reducing carbohydrates and eliminating some types altogether.

The jury is still out on whether or not this is a safe strategy from the point of view of overall health. The medical mainstream and government watchdogs of the nation's waistline have been slow to embrace this new approach. Arguments rage among so-called experts. A small handful of scientific studies is competing with a chorus of personal testimonials boasting quick and easy weight loss, coupled with plummeting cholesterol and blood pressure readings.

Conventional wisdom says that if there were a single right answer to the problem of being overweight and the health risks that go along with it, there would not be so many different diets. And if any of them really worked over the long term, there would not be so many people suffering from obesity and ill health. The best approach, therefore, must be not simply "going on a diet," but thinking about food in an entirely new way, a way that will serve as a guide to eating throughout a long and healthy life.

Carb-Conscious Diets

Here are some of the more popular carb-cutting plans:

▶ The Atkins Diet
▶ The Carbohydrate Addict's Diet
▶ The Fat Flush Plan
▶ The Glucose Revolution
▶ Protein Power
▶ The South Beach Diet
▶ Stone Age Diets (Cave Man, Paleolithic, Neanderthin, and more)
▶ Sugar Busters!
▶ The Zone

A Growing Health Threat

Unless you have been living on another planet, you surely know that America is facing an epidemic of obesity. More Americans are overweight than ever before in history, and a new generation is being raised that weighs more than it should and faces a long list of health risks that will extend beyond their growing years and into adulthood. What a terrible model we are giving our children and what a terrible legacy we are leaving them…

What does it mean if you are overweight? First, it means that you have a lot of company. According to the latest government statistics, 64 percent of American adults aged twenty years and over are overweight or obese. Forty years ago, fewer than 45 percent of adults in that age group were overweight. Among children, 15 percent of those aged twelve to nineteen years—and an equal percentage of those between the ages of six and eleven—are overweight, compared to less than 5 percent forty years ago.

But, more important than all these facts and figures, being overweight means that you are at risk for many diseases and conditions that threaten your health and may ultimately shorten your life.

Overweight in America

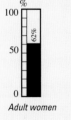
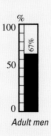
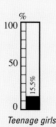
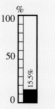
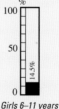
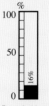

| Adult women | Adult men | Teenage girls | Teenage boys | Girls 6–11 years | Boys 6–11 years |

Bars: Adult women 62%; Adult men 67%; Teenage girls 15.5%; Teenage boys 15.5%; Girls 6–11 years 14.5%; Boys 6–11 years 16%

Source: National Center for Health Statistics, 1999–2000

The Obesity Toll

Obesity is among the leading causes of preventable disease and death in America. Deaths from obesity-related causes are thought to number in the hundreds of thousands each year.

Being overweight puts additional stress on nearly all systems of the body. The skeleton has to bear more weight than normal, causing back problems and greater wear and tear on the joints—which leads to osteoarthritis. The heart and lungs have to work harder to move blood around the body, but they must do so through blood vessels that may 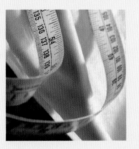 be narrowed or completely clogged with debris. Potentially fatal irregular heart rhythms are more common in people who are overweight, as is high blood pressure. Organs tend to be squeezed within the body cavity, causing indigestion, heartburn, and acid reflux (GastroEsophageal Reflux Disease, or G.E.R.D.). Circulation may be poor, resulting in varicose veins, broken capillaries, and cold hands and feet. People who are overweight tend to have poor balance and agility, and are often much less active than others. Depression, low self-esteem, social isolation, and other emotional problems are not uncommon among those whose weight is significantly above the norm.

Although there is no definitive proof, many experts believe that certain cancers are connected with being overweight—though the reasons for this are not yet understood. Some association has been found between being overweight and cancers of the breast, uterus, colon, and prostate.

Perhaps the most serious health consequence is the near certainty that a person who is overweight will develop Type 2 diabetes, a disabling disease that is the leading cause of preventable blindness in the U.S. and exists in a deadly partnership with the full spectrum of heart and circulatory diseases.

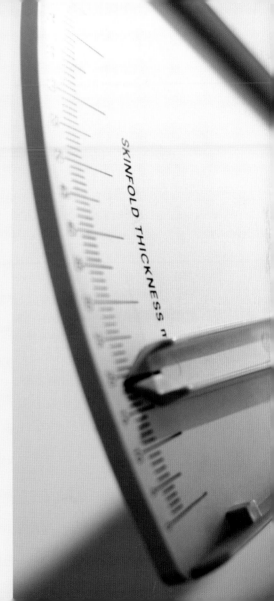

SKINFOLD THICKNESS

The scales tell the tale—excess stored fat means many health risks.

Is Dieting the Answer?

For years, people who were overweight have been told to "go on a diet" until their weight is normal for their size and height, and then to stay at that weight. Weight-reduction diets have been tried by people ranging from the extremely obese to the slightly overweight; by many people who would simply like to weigh less or fit into a favorite outfit for a special occasion; and by others whose weight is normal or even below normal, but who have a distorted sense of how their appearance compares to an unrealistic ideal.

The trouble is, "going on a diet" is a time-limited project, not a change of lifestyle—and the time can be very limited indeed. Most diets are a negative experience—full of the word *no* and the burdens of counting calories, points, or grams of this or that. They separate the dieter from others, making eating out and other social situations a trial. They dominate each day, turning daytime hours into a boring round of limited meals.

Reality check: Quick weight
loss is usually followed by
rapid weight gain.

Diets that rely on calorie restriction often make people feel weak and headachy—not to mention hungry. And diets that rely on a narrow selection of foods and food types cause cravings for forbidden tastes and textures. Some diets may be downright unhealthy— eliminating vitamins, minerals, and other nutrients that the body needs, or causing the body to make substances that tax the kidneys and may be toxic.

In short, going on a diet is often quickly followed by going off of it and returning with a vengeance to the poor eating habits that caused the problem to begin with. Cravings beget cheating, which leads to self-recrimination and a sense of failure. That is why most diets end up being short-lived and unsuccessful.

Quick Fix vs. Lifelong Healthy Habits

Many experts on nutrition and fitness believe that going on a diet is not the answer to being overweight. A temporary project may be successful for a while, though more often it is not. It is hard to subject weight loss strategies to scientifically controlled trials, but surveys of the short- and long-term effectiveness of various diets have shown that some may produce dramatic results in the first three months, but by 12 months, they are all about the same. Discouragingly, many people have trouble staying on any diet for anywhere near 12 months.

It is a rare person who has gone on only one diet. Most dieters are old hands, having lost and gained the same 10 or so pounds many times by means of a parade of diets that have come down the pike.

The answer to the high rate of diet drop-out is to make changes that can be sustained over a lifetime. That means choosing food wisely and incorporating regular exercise into a daily routine, for the rest of your life. The best way to do this is to set attainable goals that are specific and realistic. It is a good idea to revisit those goals periodically, and revise them if necessary. Losing weight this way may be more gradual than what some people boast of on the latest fad diet, but it is much more likely to last. Best of all, it will contribute to your overall wellness, energy, and vitality.

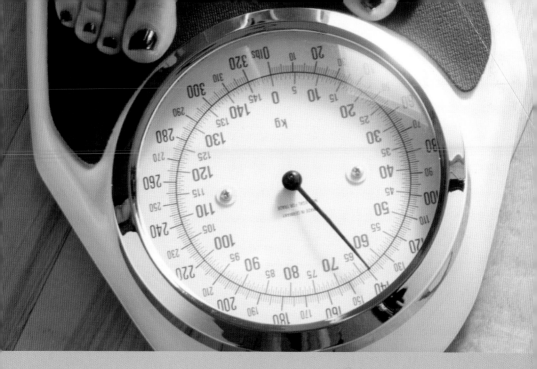

What the Experts Say...

Medical science knows a lot about how the body works—in sickness and in health. When it comes to appetite and weight loss, however, things are not so clear. In fact, much about what the body does once a morsel of food is swallowed remains a mystery second only to our murky understanding of memory, dreams, and other functions of the brain. Still, there are certain truths that have been established by solid science, proven in both the laboratory and the clinic. This is in contrast to anecdotal evidence, the wishfully convincing stories we hear about dramatic weight loss or reduction in cholesterol levels that resulted when a friend, neighbor, neighbor's friend, or relative went on this or that diet.

About Nutrition, Being Overweight, and Related Health Risks

A study of the "ecology" of American eating patterns throughout the twentieth century found a striking parallel between an increase in consumption of refined (processed) carbohydrates and a rise in the incidence of Type 2 diabetes. During that period, Americans also decreased the amount of fiber they ate while increasing their intake of high-fructose corn syrup, a sweetener that can be found in many foods and beverages—even those that do not taste particularly sweet.

The direct link between being overweight and the development of Type 2 diabetes is based on solid

Is It Chemistry?

Scientists have known about insulin's role in both health and disease for decades. More recently, researchers have found other chemicals that are manufactured by the body, and which affect feelings of hunger and satiety, as well as fat formation and levels of sugar (glucose) and fat (lipids) in the blood.

A better understanding of how these chemicals work may someday result in new drugs, or may even make it possible for the body to "medicate" itself when it comes to controlling weight and various diseases related to diet.

These are just a few of the hormone chemicals researchers are studying more closely today:

▶ **Adiponectin** is made by fat cells and secreted into the blood, where it influences how the body processes both fat and sugar. The more adiponectin, the higher the levels of high-density lipoprotein, or HDL ("good" cholesterol, *see pages 42–43*), and the lower the risk of heart attack. Low levels of the hormone, on the other hand, are often found in people who have Type 2 diabetes. Even though people who are obese have more fat cells, they produce less adiponectin.

scientific evidence. So is the close association between cardiovascular disease and this type of diabetes. The dangerous triad of being overweight, cardiovascular disease, and diabetes is not the only scientifically validated health risk, but it is increasingly common in America and other Western societies and represents the strongest reason for people to change the way they eat. The common denominator in all this is a hormone called insulin, which is secreted by special cells located in the pancreas in response to food intake. Insulin abnormalities result in diabetes (both Types 1 and 2, *see page 59*) and obesity, as well as a host of other associated health risks.

A drug that increases adiponectin production might be a boon to people with diabetes, bad cholesterol, and triglyceride numbers (*see pages 42–43*), as well as other factors that make them susceptible to a heart attack.

▶ **Ghrelin** is a hormone chemical that is secreted by the stomach, but it sends the "I'm hungry!" message to the brain. The bad news is that ghrelin secretion increases when people lose weight through diet. That might explain why cravings torment so many dieters and why it is so hard to maintain weight loss that has been achieved through diet. A drug that blocks the secretion or action of ghrelin might be the answer.

▶ **Leptin** triggers the brain to signal the body to burn calories—especially stored fat. It is part of a complex series of chemical messages that travel from the hypothalamus—the part of the brain that controls both hunger and metabolism—to the pituitary gland and from there to the thyroid, which in turn sends a message to speed up metabolism. It is less promising to use this hormone chemical in a weight-loss drug because obesity makes the body resistant to the action of leptin.

What your body does with the food you eat depends on both calorie count and type of nutrient—protein, fat, or carbohydrate. Every body needs some of each type.

About Weight Loss

Researchers know that weight loss is hard, and hardest of all for the people who need it most. Studies of people who are overweight and who either already have Type 2 diabetes or are beginning to show the signs of abnormalities in insulin activity have found that they lose less weight than people without these problems—*even when they follow exactly the same diet*.

Researchers found that low-carb/high-protein diets result in greater weight loss than those that are high-carb/low-fat, but only in the beginning. They also found that people have trouble sticking with both types of diets for long enough to maintain their weight loss. The most promising diets for people whose insulin response is abnormal emphasize high protein, moderate fat, and carbohydrates that are digested very slowly. Further studies are needed to determine whether such diets will also produce lasting weight loss and will reduce the risk of cardiovascular disease.

Regardless of the proportions of protein, fat, and carbohydrate in a given diet, most scientists cling to the "calories in/calories out" principle of weight loss: each calorie you take in is either used as fuel or stored as fat. If you take in more calories than you use, they say, you gain weight. If you use more calories than you take in, you lose weight. This is simple bookkeeping.

But is it so simple? It now looks like the body is not just an energy bank, but that its relationship with food is more interactive. Chemical reactions in the body influence how it processes, uses, and stores the energy. This does not mean that calories don't count, but that there is more to the equation than calories alone. Part of it has to do with *when* those calories are available to the body. A meal filled with sugar or refined starch simply does not stick around as long as one that is strong on protein and whole grains—so hunger returns sooner and, with it, the irresistible desire to eat more. It is also clear that the body responds to different kinds of foods in different ways.

Could It Be Magic?

Many of the low-carb/no-carb diets—and the theories on which they are based—suggest that you can eat all the fat you want and your body fat will "melt" away, so long as you do not combine it with carbohydrates. It has nothing to do with calories, these diet promoters insist. Instead, they point to something about the way the body uses food that defies logic.

Well, the truth is, there is no magic at work here. Calories still count: If you take in more energy than you burn, you will store the excess and weight gain will result. And it is still important to eat a balanced diet that includes all three major nutrients—carbohydrates, protein, and fat. Each gives the body part of what it needs to run on all cylinders.

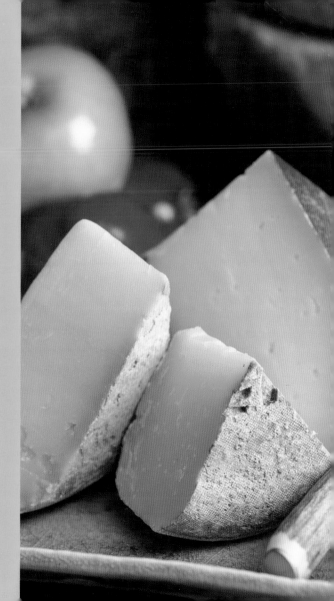

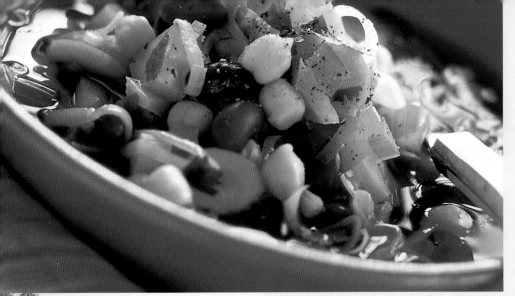

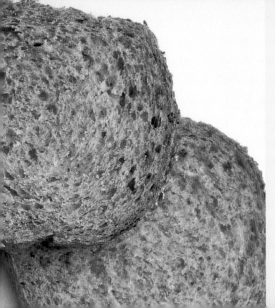

Eating the G.I. Way

Using the glycemic index as a guide to food choices is a good way to make the long-term changes needed to achieve and maintain a healthy weight, reduce the risk of health problems related to poor nutrition and being overweight, and get all the nutrients you need from a well-balanced diet. It allows you a wide range of choices without getting hung up on numbers. Best of all, it offers freedom from hunger and cravings.

Low-G.I. foods contain "slow" carbs, which take longer to be digested. They keep you feeling full because they remain intact longer, the most resistant of them still not broken down by the time they enter the small intestine. Many are naturally sweet or satisfyingly crunchy, and others offer the smooth "mouth feel" associated with the comfort foods we all crave at times, especially when we are "on a diet."

Even if you are on one of the popular low-carb diets, the G.I. will help you to be more carb-conscious. It makes sense of the rules and gives a broader dimension to the simplistic division between "good carbs" and "bad carbs."

A New Way of Thinking About Food

Even though recommendations to lower the fat content in America's diet were intended to also help people lose weight, that has not been the outcome. As fat consumption fell, carbohydrate consumption rose. After all, we all have to eat something. The problem lies in the type of carbohydrates that most of us choose to replace the fat with: starchy and sweet foods. These foods are troublemakers. They bring about changes in insulin and other hormones that make it more difficult for the body to access the fuel it needs; they also lead to overeating. Strange as it may seem, we feel less full and get hungry sooner after eating starchy and sweet foods.

Losing weight is no longer a matter of vanity; it is a matter of life and death. But if we are facing an obesity epidemic, we also have a plague of fad diets. The latest batch demonize carbohydrates, and these diets are selling like hotcakes. The glycemic index brings some sanity to the picture, offering a solid scientific basis for making smart food choices. No diet works if you don't stick to it. The beauty of using the G.I. is that it gives you a huge range of foods to choose from and does not require you to eat bird-size portions. The G.I. works *with* your body's metabolism, rather than trying to manipulate it. It allows you to follow a balanced diet and gain the health benefits of a wide range of foods. Best of all, it lowers the risk of the most serious threats to America's health: obesity, high cholesterol, high blood pressure, and Type 2 diabetes.

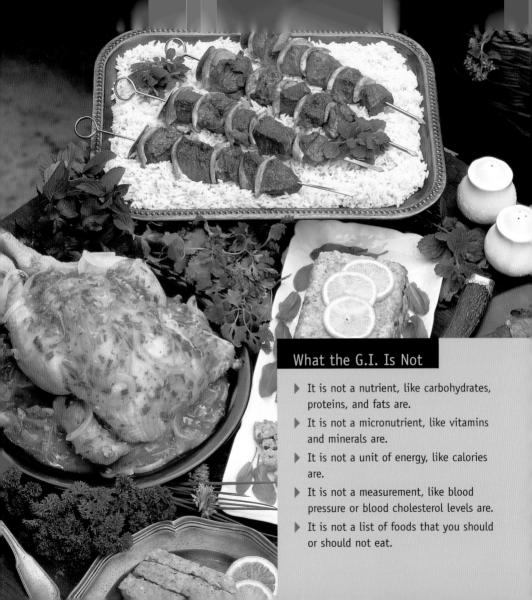

What the G.I. Is Not

▶ It is not a nutrient, like carbohydrates, proteins, and fats are.

▶ It is not a micronutrient, like vitamins and minerals are.

▶ It is not a unit of energy, like calories are.

▶ It is not a measurement, like blood pressure or blood cholesterol levels are.

▶ It is not a list of foods that you should or should not eat.

1 What Is the Glycemic Index?

In 1981, Dr. David Jenkins and colleagues in the department of nutritional sciences at the University of Toronto published a paper in *The American Journal of Clinical Nutrition* that introduced the glycemic index (G.I.), which they described as a physiological basis for classifying carbohydrate foods. That is, instead of focusing on how many or what type of carbohydrates a food contains, they were looking at how the body responds to the carbs—specifically, how quickly and by how much the blood sugar level rises within the first two hours after the food is eaten.

The Answer to an Oversimplified Message

The glycemic index was developed to help people with diabetes maintain better control over their blood sugar levels, a health- and often life-preserving matter for those with the disease. Soon, however, both the diet and food industries took notice when the glycemic index looked like something they could sell to the general public. Unfortunately, this has led to much misunderstanding, because the message was oversimplified to "Carbs are bad; avoid them altogether."

The truth is the body needs carbohydrates, but not all carbohydrates are equal. The tricky part is knowing which carbs provide needed fuel without making unreasonable demands on the metabolism. The handy part is that the glycemic index provides a simple, but scientific way to distinguish between "good" carbs and "bad" carbs. This is just as important for those who are healthy as it is for those who are suffering from diabetes and other diet-related disorders.

Life is a banquet, but what should you choose to eat? The answer lies in the glycemic index.

Metabolism in Brief

Metabolism is the name given to everything the body does to process and use ingested material to build, maintain, and repair cells, tissues, and organs, as well as to fuel activity. In short, it is the engine that keeps the body running.

One of the most important aspects of metabolism relates to the digestion, absorption, use, and storage of the food we eat. It operates with the help of hormones and the glands that secrete them; with the assistance of the full length of the digestive tract and the chemical and physical activities that take place within it; and with the aid of the bloodstream, which carries processed nutrients to the cells that need them.

Each of the major nutrients—carbohydrate, protein, and fat—is broken down and rearranged into forms the body can use. Also known as macronutrients, they are absolutely essential to the operation of the body. You could not live long without any of them.

When carbohydrates are digested, they are transformed into glucose, which is a type of sugar. Glucose is absorbed into the bloodstream, where it has a profound effect on many operations of the human body. Among other things, glucose is the most readily available fuel for energy and the brain's main source of nutrition.

Let me repeat that: Glucose is the brain's main source of nutrition. *Without carbohydrates, the body must look elsewhere for glucose to feed the brain.*

The breakdown of some carbohydrates begins even before they reach the stomach, dissolving in the mouth and entering the bloodstream through the membranes that line the mouth, throat, and esophagus. Most are digested in the stomach, but others are still intact when they arrive in the small intestine. These last are termed resistant starches. Depending on the type of carbohydrate eaten, glucose may turn up in the blood quickly and in a huge torrent, or slowly and gradually. As we will see, slowly and gradually is the better way.

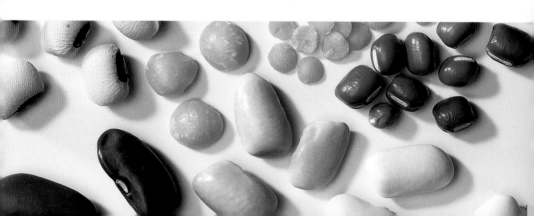

When Metabolism Bites Back

Glucose, or blood sugar, is just a passerby in the bloodstream, on its way to be stored or used for energy. The level of blood sugar rises soon after food is eaten and then subsides. When the body is unable to clear glucose efficiently, it remains in the blood for too long or at levels that are too high. This causes a great deal of damage throughout the body.

Here is a list of the most common diseases or disorders related to glucose metabolism:

▶ **Type 1 diabetes:** an autoimmune disease that damages or destroys the insulin-producing cells of the pancreas, resulting in destructively high blood sugar levels.

▶ **Type 2 diabetes:** a disease in which insulin secretion cannot control blood sugar levels—because there is not enough insulin or it is not strong enough, or both.

▶ **Hypoglycemia:** abnormally low blood sugar levels; it may result from many causes, including abnormal fluctuations in insulin secretion.

▶ **Impaired glucose tolerance:** a prediabetic state in which blood glucose levels are higher than normal, but have not yet reached the diabetes threshold.

▶ **Insulin exhaustion:** depletion of insulin or reduction in the number or activity of the cells that manufacture it; may occur after a prolonged period of excessive demand.

▶ **Metabolic syndrome:** also called *Syndrome X* and *insulin resistance syndrome*. A group of disorders—including obesity, abnormal cholesterol levels, and high blood pressure, along with insufficient or inefficient insulin activity—that increase the risk of developing, and even dying from, cardiovascular disease, Type 2 diabetes, and stroke.

They may seem unrelated, but both diabetes and cardiovascular disease are linked to impaired glucose metabolism.

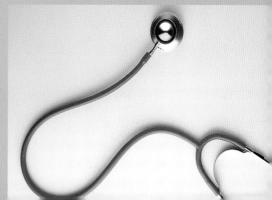

Use It or Store It

Unlike carbohydrates, fats are not reduced to glucose, and proteins are only when there is no other choice. Instead, fats are broken down into fatty acids and proteins into amino acids. All three of these breakdown products are then packaged according to when they are needed and what they are needed for.

Each product has several forms, some for use and some for storage. Some fatty acids are made into hormones and other chemicals that the body uses, but most are bundled as triglycerides and carried through the blood to be stored in fat cells, where they simply wait until they are needed to provide energy. The fat in these storage depots insulates the body and cushions organs.

Glucose can be used immediately to provide energy (to run the body or to fuel activity, for instance), or it can be stored in the liver and muscle cells as glycogen. When it is required for energy, the glycogen is converted back to glucose and burned as fuel. If all the storage space in the liver and muscles is filled, then the excess will be sent to the fat cells. The same is true for amino acids, which are used to manufacture and repair cells of all kinds, including those that make up the muscles, the skeleton, and the immune system. In a pinch, they can be used to make glucose. Whatever is not needed right away is stored.

Although the liver and muscles can store only a limited amount of glycogen—about 100 grams in the liver and 400 grams in the muscles—fat cells have a relatively large storage capacity; when that is filled, more fat cells are easily made. And that, of course, is where the problem lies. Eat more of any of the three macronutrients than your body needs, and the leftovers will be deposited in an endlessly expandable fat bank. In other words, you will get fat and then fatter.

Glucose supplies the energy, while amino acids provide the materials to build muscles as well as to repair them.

How It Works

Carbohydrate →	Glucose →	Liver →	storage (as glycogen) triglyceride synthesis (excess)
	→	Other tissues	
		→ Brain and kidney →	energy production
		→ Muscle →	storage predominantly (as glycogen)
Protein →	Amino acids →	Liver →	energy production (& protein synthesis)
	→	Other tissues →	protein synthesis
Fat →	Fatty acids →	Fat cells →	storage (triglycerides)
	→	Muscle →	energy production (small amount)

Whether protein, fat, or carbohydrate, everything you eat is converted to a form your body can either use or store.

Scientifically Speaking

The glycemic index represents a scientific way of measuring how quickly the body processes the carbohydrates in food, transforming them into glucose, which then goes into the bloodstream. This is called the postprandial ("after meal") glycemic response. The G.I. is determined by measuring and graphing the level of glucose in the blood as it rises and then falls over the course of the first two hours after consumption of 50 grams of a given carbohydrate and then comparing it to the increase caused by 50 grams of pure glucose in the same person over the same length of time.

Pure glucose is the *index* or *reference* food. Some laboratories use 50 grams of white bread as the index food. Because everyone's metabolism is different, foods are tested multiple times with different subjects—some with normal metabolisms, some with diabetes—and the results are averaged according to a formula more complicated than most of us need to know about.

The index food—whether it is glucose or white bread—always has a G.I. of 100. The test food's G.I. is always a comparison with that index food. For example, cornflakes have a G.I. of 84, which means that a serving containing 50 grams of carbohydrate (**not** 50 grams of cornflakes) delivers glucose to the blood only slightly less rapidly than 50 grams of pure glucose. This would be considered a high-G.I. food. In contrast, a serving of oatmeal containing 50 grams of carbohydrate has a G.I. of 49, which is in the low-G.I. range.

Fats and proteins have very little effect on blood sugar levels—for all practical purposes, none. Because the G.I. quantifies the glycemic response, only carbohydrates are measured.

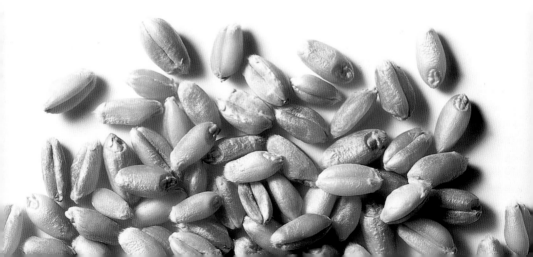

The nutrient content of a specific food—that is, the amount of protein, fat, and carbohydrate it contains—and the amount of energy (calories) it provides can be measured in a laboratory using relatively simple methods. The outcome will always be the same.

How the body uses that food, however, depends on many variables, including any given individual's age, metabolic rate, level of activity, body composition, and, perhaps most important of all, state of health.

People with diabetes and other metabolic abnormalities do not process food as efficiently as those whose health is normal. Many other people who appear to be in good health may have unrecognized prediabetic conditions that impair their ability to process, use, and store nutrients. That is why the G.I. of foods is based on an average glycemic response by more than one test subject. It is also one of the main reasons why, on a day-to-day basis, it makes sense to use G.I. *ranges*—low, medium, and high—rather than specific G.I. numbers.

Effects on Blood Sugar Levels

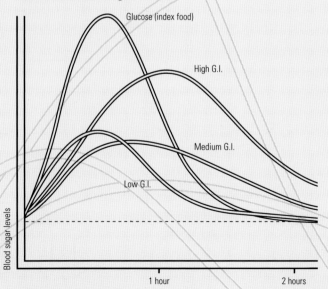

Glucose (index food)

High G.I.

Medium G.I.

Low G.I.

Blood sugar levels

1 hour   2 hours

The effect on blood sugar levels of glucose compared to high-, medium-, and low-G.I. foods.

G.I. Ranges

Less than 5 = none

5–55 = low

56–70 = medium

More than 70 = high

What Is the Glycemic Index?

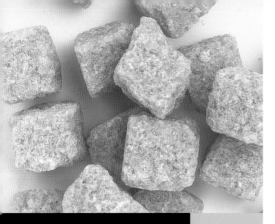

From Starch to Sugar

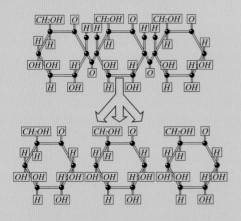

Glucose, the form of sugar found in the blood, is made of a single CHO molecule ($C_6H_{12}O_6$). When digested, starch molecules are broken up into many glucose molecules.

Whether simple or complex, all carbohydrates consist of carbon, hydrogen, and oxygen.

Spotlight on Sugars

Why is there sugar in your blood even when you haven't eaten any? The answer has to do with the molecular makeup of all carbohydrates: carbon, hydrogen, and oxygen (CHO). Glucose is the simplest type of carbohydrate, comprising a single CHO molecule made up of six atoms of carbon, 12 of hydrogen, and six more of oxygen—$C_6H_{12}O_6$. All carbohydrates, no matter how complex they are, end up as glucose by the time they are fully digested.

It's in Your Blood

Your body is a sophisticated energy refinery. Parts of it grind up food while other parts secrete chemicals to dissolve it. As the food progresses through the full length of the digestive system, nutrients are separated from waste. The nutrients are absorbed into the blood, which carries them throughout the body, dropping off bundles in various places for further processing, storage, or use.

Fats travel in the bloodstream as complex molecules called triglycerides; proteins travel as extremely complex molecules called amino acids. Carbohydrates travel as simple glucose molecules. When it is needed to supply immediate energy, the glucose is simply burned. Anything that is not needed right away is turned into glycogen and stored in the liver and muscles, with the excess going into the fat cells.

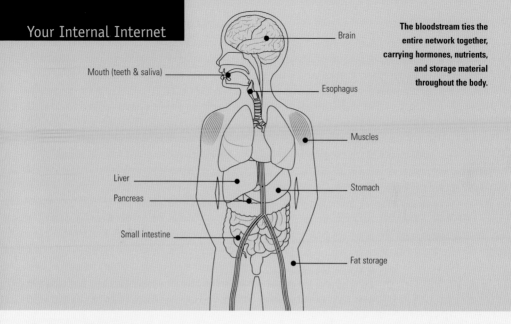

Brain

Mouth (teeth & saliva)

Esophagus

Muscles

Liver

Stomach

Pancreas

Small intestine

Fat storage

The bloodstream ties the entire network together, carrying hormones, nutrients, and storage material throughout the body.

The Master Hormone

When most people hear the word *insulin* they think about diabetes. They may not know what insulin does, just that it is something that people with diabetes have trouble with. In fact, insulin is the stage manager of our metabolism. We all need it, and we manufacture it on demand.

Insulin is made by specialized "islet" cells of the pancreas, which secretes it into the bloodstream in response to the presence of glucose. Insulin's job is to send glucose on its way for immediate use or for further processing and storage. One of the many things insulin does is activate an enzyme that helps convert glucose to storable fat. Another is to increase the activity of a different enzyme, which promotes the storage of fat. Insulin also inhibits the activity of a third enzyme, which breaks down stored fat and prepares it for use.

These fat-storing activities hint at a good reason why people who want to lose weight should keep insulin secretion at low levels. The only way to do that is to reduce the demand for insulin, and the way to do that is to eat foods that produce a low and slow postprandial glycemic response. In short: foods that have a low G.I. number.

What Is the Glycemic Index?

The Carbs Have It

You have probably heard about *simple* and *complex* carbohydrates. But what do these terms mean? They really just describe molecular structure. As has been said before, all carbohydrates consist of carbon, hydrogen, and oxygen (CHO), but the number and arrangement of the molecules vary. The simpler the molecular structure, the more quickly it can be broken down and made available to the body. More complicated molecular structures are harder to disassemble, so it takes longer for the nutrients they contain to be packaged for use by the body.

When it comes to carbohydrates (*see pages 34–35*), sugars have the least complex molecular structure, so they are digested and transformed into glucose quickly. Starch molecules are more complex. Of the two types of starch molecules, amylopectin is processed into glucose more quickly than amylose. Most complex of all is fiber. In fact, it is so complex that the digestive system cannot disassemble it at all.

That's really what's behind the "good" carbs and "bad" carbs idea. You can think of low-G.I. foods as resembling those "sustained-release" capsules that deliver small amounts of medicine to your system over the course of hours. Carbohydrates that are digested and absorbed slowly have low G.I. ratings because glucose is released into the blood gradually, resulting in a slow, moderate release of insulin in response. That's what makes them "good." Carbohydrates that are digested and absorbed quickly, causing a spike in blood glucose levels and requiring a rush of insulin, have high G.I. ratings and earn the label "bad."

Many fruits contain more than one of the three carbohydrate types: sugar, starch, and fiber.

What Is a Carbohydrate?

A carbohydrate is one of the three macronutrient components of food. Carbohydrate is our main source of energy—providing about 80 percent of the body's fuel needs—and the only nutrient the brain can use. Sugars and starches are digestible carbohydrates, which have 4 calories per gram. Fiber is indigestible by humans, so it provides no calories at all.

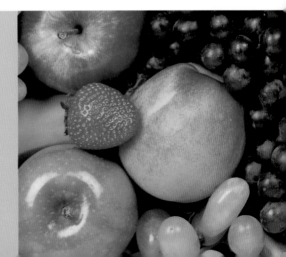

It Takes All Kinds

It is important to realize that few foods contain only one type of carbohydrate. Table sugar and other sweeteners are exceptions: they are all made of those simple, easy-to-digest molecules. That's why people get "sugar highs" from them. Fruit, however, contains both sugar (in the form of fructose) and fiber, and some fruits contain a lot of fiber. Plums and apricots (both fresh and dried), and pears are good examples. Bananas contain both sugar and starch; as they ripen, they become sweeter and less starchy. Starchy foods typically contain more than one kind of starch, some being more readily digestible than others. The miscellaneous nature of carb content gets even more complicated in prepared foods. Bread is a prime example. Look at the ingredient list on any package of bread: each ingredient is digested at its own rate and produces its own glycemic response.

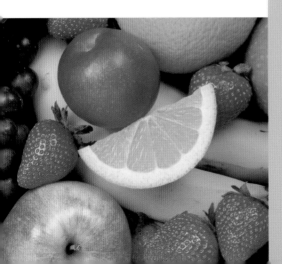

"Natural" Whole Grain Bread? A Reading Lesson

Here's an ingredient list on a randomly chosen loaf of supermarket bread. The order of ingredients reflects the amount of each, starting with the highest. Except for a bit of fat and a smidgen of protein, it's all carbs all the time.

▶ Stone ground 100% whole-wheat flour
▶ Water
▶ Rye meal
▶ Wheat gluten
▶ Crushed wheat
▶ Vegetable oil
▶ Raisin juice concentrate
▶ Oats
▶ High fructose corn syrup
▶ Molasses
▶ Yeast

Plus 2% or less of the following: honey, rye flakes, salt, coarse corn, kibbled barley, kibbled rye, kibbled triticale, vinegar, modified soy lecithin, cultured whey, rice bran, unbleached wheat flour, ground amaranth, ground buckwheat, ground millet.

Can you pick out the sugars, starches, and fiber-rich ingredients? Your digestive system can.

Carb Categories

All carbohydrates are saccharides, which basically consist of one or more glucose molecules arranged in chains. Sugars have the shortest and least complex chains; saccharide chains that make up starches and fiber can be very long and complex.

The acidity of citrus fruit lowers the G.I. total when added to other foods.

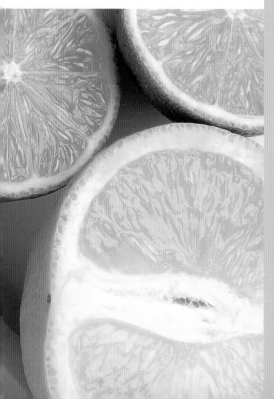

Saccharides

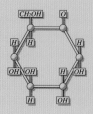

Monosaccharides

These sugars have only one molecule.

▶ Glucose—the sugar found in your blood; also used to sweeten foods

▶ Fructose—fruit sugar

▶ Galactose—combines with glucose to form lactose

▶ Dextrose—also called invert sugar; found in starches

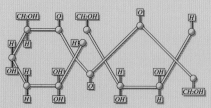

Disaccharides

These sugars have two molecules, but are still very simple and easy to break down.

▶ Sucrose—table sugar

▶ Lactose—found in milk

▶ Maltose—found in starches, especially malt

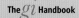

Polysaccharides

These are the complex carbohydrates: starches, fiber, and other substances that are added to food. You may find them by name on food labels or they may be listed as "other carbohydrates."

texture; some modified starches are gummy, others gooey, some add bulk, others stand up well to heat.

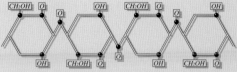

Dietary Fibers

These non-starch polysaccharides are so complex that humans cannot break them down into glucose, so they have no effect on blood sugar levels and thus earn a "no G.I." rating.

- Cellulose—insoluble fiber found in many fruits, vegetables, legumes, and grains
- Pectin—soluble fiber found in many fruits
- Gum—soluble fiber used to thicken, bind, or give food a smooth texture; examples include guar, acacia, and arabic

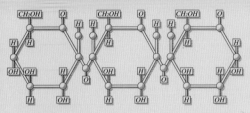

Starches

- Amylopectin—one of the two kinds of starch found in food; its branching molecular structure makes it relatively easy to digest. Foods that have a greater proportion of amylopectin have a higher G.I. rating than those with more amylose.

- Amylose—the other kind of food starch; because its molecular structure is more compact than that of amylopectin, it is digested more slowly. Foods that have a greater proportion of amylose have a lower G.I. rating.

- Maltodextrin—a sweet food additive made from cornstarch.

- Modified starch—various molecules manipulated to alter their behavior or

Sugar Alcohols

Also called polyols, these are the "no sugar added" food sweeteners. Though technically carbohydrates, they are incompletely metabolized, yielding far fewer calories than sugar. Most, but not all, have little effect on blood sugar unless consumed in quantity, potentially a problem for people with diabetes.

- Glycerol (glycerin)
- Maltitol
- Mannitol
- Sorbitol
- Xylitol

G.I. Levels

Choose your daily carb quotient from low- and medium-G.I. foods. In general:

▶ **Low G.I.** = non-starchy fruits and vegetables.

▶ **Medium G.I.** = legumes (peas, beans, lentils) and whole unprocessed cereals and grains.

▶ **High G.I.** = potatoes and refined grains, cereals, and flours.

But there are some surprises. Read on to find out how and why you can include some sugars and pastas in your life, and what foods you can eat as much of as you wish.

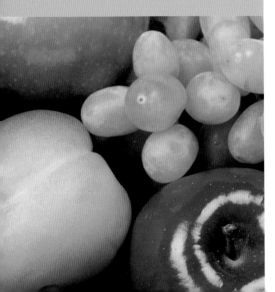

Very good carbs: Apples, peaches, and grapes are low-G.I., high-fiber, and vitamin-rich.

How Many Carbs Do You Need?

The minimum amount of carbohydrates any adult needs is 150 grams a day. Less than that will, over time, starve the muscles and brain. As a last resort, glycogen stores in the liver and muscles can make up the shortfall, but it's a temporary solution, at best.

Most nutrition experts recommend that 55 percent of a person's daily calorie intake should be carbohydrates. If you regularly consume 2,000 calories, for example, 1,100 of them should come from carbohydrates. That's 275 grams.

These recommendations do not distinguish between "good" and "bad" carbs or a food's G.I. But you should make the distinction, especially if you need to lose weight or are under a doctor's care because you have diabetes, a prediabetic condition, high blood pressure, high cholesterol, clogged arteries or other heart problems.

Fiber: The G.I.-Free Carb

My grandmother called it roughage and she encouraged me to eat my apple's skin, flesh, and core, and to pull out and eat the membrane from my half grapefruit after I'd scooped up the juicy sections in between. She may not have known why, but Grandma was on to something. What she was advising me to eat is fiber, an amazing food component that has no calories but offers many health benefits. Like water, that other no-cal miracle, fiber is something most of us don't get enough of.

When it comes to calories—as well as glycemic response—fiber is a big fat zero. Even though it is a carbohydrate, it passes through the body without contributing any nutrients and having no effect on blood glucose levels. Fiber does not *lower* the G.I. of foods; it just doesn't count. All the same, it performs many valuable services.

Fiber is either soluble, absorbing liquid to become a gummy or gel-like mass, or insoluble, retaining its form as it passes through the digestive tract. Because both kinds of fiber are indigestible, they stick around for a long time, making you feel fuller for longer.

Insoluble fiber adds bulk and texture to food, and helps to move waste through the colon more quickly. There is no question that it promotes bowel regularity and helps prevent constipation and a painful condition called *diverticulosis*, but it may also protect against colon cancer. Soluble fiber, also called viscous fiber, adds bulk and a pleasant "mouth feel." Even more important, it also slows the absorption of other carbohydrates.

Fiber is found in many foods. The obvious ones are whole grains and cereals, but many fruits contain a soluble fiber called pectin. To get the most out of a piece of fruit, wash it well so you can eat the skin. Peel citrus fruit, but eat the membrane between sections. Fruit juice is *not* a source of fiber. Salad and other leafy green vegetables are though, since they contain little more than cellulose, an insoluble fiber. They have virtually no calories, but plenty of vitamins and minerals, and a lot of bulk and crunch. Oats, barley, and other cereal grains contain soluble fiber. Dried beans are a treasure trove of both soluble and insoluble fibers, and are universally low-G.I. foods.

The healthiest diet is based on "traditional foods": dense, grainy breads, oatmeal, stews, casseroles, and other dishes made with whole grains, dried beans, low-G.I. pasta and rice, and nonstarchy vegetables.

Find the Fiber

Try to include at least 25–30 grams of fiber in your daily diet. It's easy if you choose these fiber-rich foods:

▶ Whole grains: especially oats, barley, and rye

▶ Bran: oat and wheat

▶ High-fiber breakfast cereals

▶ Seeds: pumpkin, sunflower, sesame

▶ Nuts

▶ Dried beans and legumes

▶ Fruit: apples, pears, peaches, plums, citrus, grapes, prunes; eat them whole, since juices lack fiber and are much higher on the G.I.

▶ Salad and other green vegetables

Energy Is What You Eat

Even though fat and protein do not contribute to the glucose response and so are not part of the glycemic index, no discussion of choosing what to eat would be complete without brief mention of the two other macronutrients. Like carbohydrates, fat and protein are absolutely essential to health and life. All provide fuel for the body. When burned, they release energy that can be used for a range of activities: voluntary (movement and exercise) and involuntary (the ongoing processes that keep your body running).

Fat and protein are often found in combination, especially in dairy products and other foods of animal origin.

What Is a Calorie?

A calorie is a unit of heat, which is really just a way to measure energy. In the case of food, it tells you how much potential energy it contains. When used, it will produce heat. One calorie is the amount of heat required to raise the temperature of one gram of water by one degree centigrade (a little over half a degree Fahrenheit).

How Much Energy?

As an energy source, fat provides more than double what protein and carbohydrates do. Sounds like a good thing? Let's put it another way: Every gram of fat contains 9 calories, whereas protein and carbohydrates each contain only 4 calories per gram.

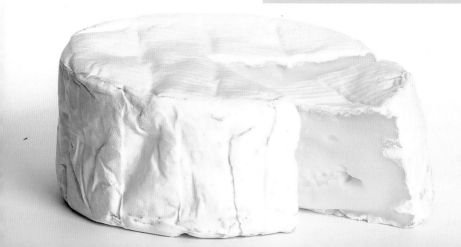

Alcohol is not, strictly speaking, a macronutrient. Each gram of alcohol has 7 calories, but it is not used by the body as a source of energy, nor does it supply what the body needs. To the contrary, alcohol may contribute to malnutrition, not only because it interferes with the absorption of some important micronutrients, but also because people who drink in excess may forget to eat. On the other hand, it loosens inhibitions, which may lead to mindless munching. One factor, of course, is what you drink. Some studies suggest that red wine contains nonalcoholic substances that may promote health, so a 5-ounce glass of wine a day is sometimes recommended. Beer, on the other hand, contains a lot of carbs to go with the calories. The new "low-carb" beers are nothing more than "lite" or "near" beers repackaged to take advantage of the low-carb trend. Sweet wines, liqueurs, and many mixed drinks are chock full of sugar.

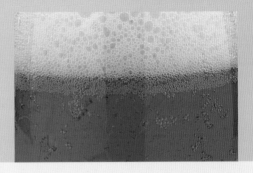

It may have calories—7 per gram, to be precise—but alcohol is not a nutrient.

Fellow Travelers: Fat and Protein

You can find fat riding solo in vegetable oils and butter, but most often it is found with protein, and specifically with protein from animal sources. From a well-marbled steak to a fresh egg, an oozing wedge of soft cheese to a crisp-skinned piece of broiled chicken, fat and protein go together like a hand in a glove. This makes it difficult to eat a high-protein diet without also consuming quite a bit of fat, and, along with it, taking in more than twice the calories (gram for gram) that protein and carbohydrates provide.

Good Fat, Bad Fat, and Very Bad Fat

We do need some fat in our diets because our bodies use it for many different functions, but none of us needs as much fat as we actually consume. What makes the subject so confusing is that some fats are better for us than others, and some fats are so bad for us that we should not be eating them at all. Unfortunately, those very bad fats are found on the shelves of every supermarket aisle—except, of course, for the ones featuring laundry detergent and paper plates!

Like the different types of carbohydrate, fat types are grouped according to molecular structure. The two broad groupings of fats are saturated and unsaturated fats.

The term *saturation* refers to the number of hydrogen atoms bonded to carbon atoms in a fat molecule. In saturated fats, all the carbon–hydrogen links are filled. Unsaturated fats have some carbon–hydrogen links, but other carbon atoms do not have a dance partner.

That doesn't mean you have to subject any fat you might consider eating to molecular analysis—though your body can and does. A simpler way to look at it is that saturated fats are solid at room temperature whereas unsaturated fats are liquid. According to that rule, butter and the fat that clings to chicken skin and surrounds steaks and chops are all saturated. Oils are unsaturated.

Within the unsaturated category are mono-unsaturated and polyunsaturated fats. Again, this

Fat Types

▶ **Saturated:** solid at room temperature; comes mostly from animal sources.

▶ **Unsaturated:** Oils; liquid at room temperature; comes mostly from plant sources; may be monounsaturated or polyunsaturated.

▶ **Trans fats:** short for *trans fatty acids*; also called *hydrogenated* and *partially hydrogenated*; oils that have been artificially saturated with hydrogen to produce a solid fat.

How Much Fat Do You Need?

Many low-carb diets are, by default, high in fat. After all, if you are eating fewer carbs but not starving yourself, you must be eating more protein and, with it, more fat. It is a mistake to think that it doesn't matter how much fat you eat as long as you cut the carbs. Remember, calories count. Take in more than you use and your body will turn the excess into fat.

Recommendations for daily fat intake range from the very low—2 percent of total calories—to no more than 30 percent. No matter where in that range they fall, all say you should eat fewer saturated fats and more unsaturated ones. As a rule of thumb, no more than one-third of the fat you eat should be saturated.

refers to how many unbonded carbon atoms the molecule contains: monounsaturated fats have room for one more hydrogen atom; polyunsaturated fats have room for two or more. And then there are trans fats, an evil mutant produced when unsaturated fats are subjected to a manufacturing process called hydrogenation, which adds hydrogen atoms to fill some or all of the empty linkages. Anything that is called hydrogenated and partially hydrogenated is a trans fat.

In some ways, saturated fat can be thought of as "bad" and unsaturated fat as "good." In truth, most fats and oils are mixtures of the two types, but are grouped according to the type they contain the most of. Like their carb cousins, it all has to do with what happens when they get into the body. To understand that, we have to know more about the cholesterol twins—high-density lipoprotein (HDL, the "good" twin) and low-density lipoprotein (LDL, the "bad" twin)—and LDL's mischievous pal, triglycerides.

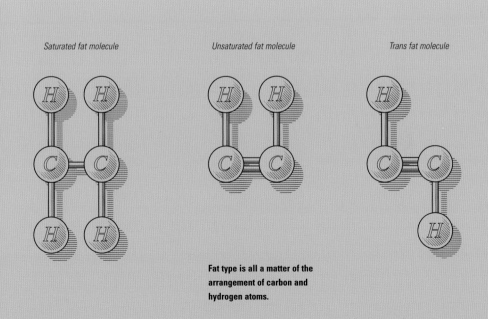

Saturated fat molecule *Unsaturated fat molecule* *Trans fat molecule*

Fat type is all a matter of the arrangement of carbon and hydrogen atoms.

Clearing Up Cholesterol Confusion

One of the most confusing things about fat is the difference between the fat we eat (dietary fat) and the fat in our bodies. You already know that you don't have to eat fat to get fat. Your body can make fat out of any of the three macronutrients. The same is true of cholesterol.

People tend to think that cholesterol is a kind of fat that comes from food. Although it is true that some foods contain cholesterol, and those foods tend also to be high in fat, cholesterol is not a fat and most of the cholesterol in your body is made by your body itself. And though cholesterol is generally thought of as a bad thing, your body makes it for a reason. This waxy substance is an ingredient in many hormones. It makes some digestive chemicals and helps convert vitamin D to a usable form for building

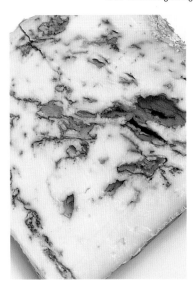

bones. Cholesterol is also used to construct cell membranes and brain and nerve tissue. It sure sounds like great stuff, doesn't it? It is what is left over, however, that causes the problems. Carried in the blood, "bad" cholesterol clogs arteries and contributes to heart attacks, strokes, and other serious threats to your health.

A Lipid Lesson

Cholesterol is carried in the blood in molecular packages called lipoproteins, which, as the name suggests, are a sort of fat-protein hybrid. There are several types, but the ones we're concerned with are high-density and low-density lipoproteins, or HDL and LDL. Without getting too technical:

LDL is referred to as "bad cholesterol" because, as it travels from the liver to other parts of the body that need it, it tends to form the artery-clogging clumps that cause cardiovascular disease. So the lower your LDL is, the better.

HDL is referred to as "good cholesterol" because it removes excess cholesterol from the blood and carries it back to the liver for reprocessing. So the higher your HDL, the better.

Triglyceride is a fat-transport molecule that is sometimes included in the "cholesterol count," even though it does not actually contain cholesterol. Like LDL, triglyceride is associated with clogged arteries and cardiovascular disease, and high levels of triglycerides in the body are a red flag for diabetes. So the lower your triglycerides, the better for your overall health.

The New Numbers

Every few years, the guardians of America's health revise the yardstick for measuring cholesterol levels. Cholesterol-lowering drugs (statins) are recommended for high-risk people who don't meet these guidelines:

▶ LDL

Under 100	Optimal
100–129	Near optimal
130–159	Borderline high
160–189	High
Over 190	Very high

▶ HDL

Under 40	Low
Over 60	High

▶ Total Cholesterol (LDL + HDL)

Under 200	Desirable
200–239	Borderline high
Over 240	High

▶ Triglycerides

Under 150	Normal
150–199	Borderline high
200–499	High
500 or more	Very high

How do you measure up? If you do not know your cholesterol numbers, ask your doctor about getting them checked.

Source: ATP III Guidelines, National Cholesterol Education Program, 2001

That brings us back to the fats we eat: saturated fats raise LDL levels, trans fats do that *plus* lower HDL, whereas unsaturated fats lower LDL. That's why you should try to eat more unsaturated fat and less saturated fat, and avoid trans fats all together. It's easy to do if you know where to find each kind.

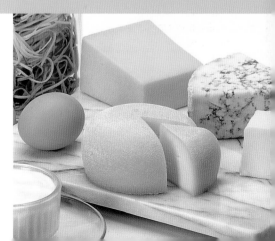

Delicious as they are, cheese, eggs, and other dairy foods contain saturated fat.

What Is the Glycemic Index?

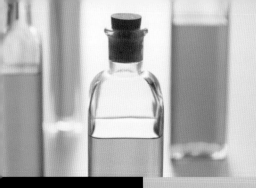

Good Fat: Where to Find It

Unsaturated fats contain Omega-3 fatty acids, which many experts think enhance cardiovascular health and lower heart attack risk. Try to get two-thirds of your daily fat allowance from unsaturated fats, but remember that even "good" fats contain 9 calories per gram, or approximately 45 calories per teaspoon.

Sources of Fat

Monounsaturated Oils

▶ Canola (also called rapeseed oil)
▶ Nut oils: almond, walnut, hazelnut, etc.
▶ Olive
▶ Peanut

Fish Oils

Most fish oils are primarily unsaturated fats, some more mono, some more poly. They contain a type of fatty acid called Omega-3, which has many health benefits. Fish oils by themselves are quite unpalatable, so the best way to get them is to eat a few servings of fatty fish—salmon, mackerel, lake trout, herring, sardines, and tuna—each week.

Polyunsaturated Oils

▶ Corn
▶ Cottonseed
▶ Flaxseed
▶ Grapeseed
▶ Safflower
▶ Sesame (really closer to half mono and half poly)
▶ Soybean
▶ Sunflower
▶ Vegetable (often called blended vegetable oil)

Both fish and vegetable oils contain Omega-3 fatty acids. Flaxseed oil is a particularly rich source.

The *gi* Handbook

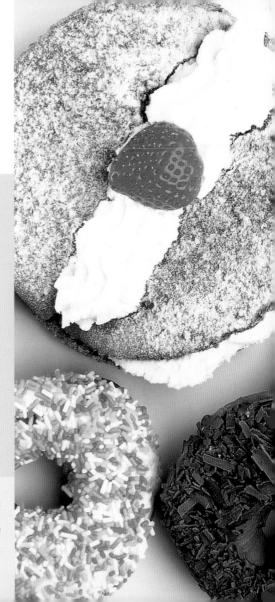

Bad Fat: How to Avoid It

Limit saturated fats to no more than one-third of your daily fat allowance. Saturated fats are found mostly in meat and other animal products, with three exceptions. Although they are from plant sources, coconut, palm, and palm kernel oils contain a high percentage of saturated fat.

Here are some common sources of saturated fat:

▶ Meat: beef, veal, pork, lamb
▶ Organ meats: liver, kidneys, brains, sweetbreads
▶ Deli and luncheon meats
▶ Eggs
▶ Cream
▶ Whole milk
▶ Cheese
▶ Baked goods and mixes: many have lard or palm, palm kernel, or coconut oil

There are lots of reasons to avoid these goodies: lots of sugar, lots of saturated and trans fats.

What Is the Glycemic Index?

The Truth About Trans Fat

At first, hydrogenation seemed like a boon to food manufacturers and consumers alike. Someone thought it would be a terrific idea to modify liquid fat so it would take on solid form at room temperature. *Voilà*: margarine. Better yet, adding this kind of fat to baked goods keeps them fresher longer. And then there's "mouth feel": hydrogenated fats give many foods a nice creamy texture that you can't normally get without adding a ton of cream—which is full of globules of saturated fat.

The trouble is, after trans fats found their way into our cookies and canned soups, our crackers and sauces, our breakfast bars and french fries, researchers discovered that their harmful effect on the body was greater even than those of saturated fats. That is particularly bad news considering how much trans fat is in the foods that most of us eat. Like saturated fats, trans fats raise LDL levels and increase insulin resistance, but they also lower HDL levels and raise triglycerides—a sure-fire recipe for heart disease.

Very Bad Fat: Where It's Hiding

Trans fats have been called "stealth" fats because for years manufacturers were not required to identify them on food labels. As of January 1, 2006, all food labels in the U.S. have to list trans fat content by grams. Many food manufacturers have already started doing so.

Happily, many have also stopped using as much trans fat in their products—but you still need to read the label. If you don't see trans fats listed in the "nutrition facts" panel, check the ingredient list for the words *hydrogenated* and *partially hydrogenated*.

Read the label, and just say no to trans fats.

Here are some notorious trans fat traps:

▶ Breakfast cereals
▶ Stick margarine
▶ Solid vegetable shortening
▶ Crackers
▶ Cookies
▶ Snack foods: chips, pretzels, "butter-flavored" popcorn, etc.
▶ Taco shells and chips
▶ Creamy salad dressings
▶ Baking mixes
▶ Packaged frostings and icings
▶ Frozen cakes and pastries
▶ Donuts
▶ Fast foods of every type

The Protein Portion

Protein is more important to human nutrition than is implied by the amount of space allotted to it here. Like fat, it is not included in the G.I. because it has a minimal effect on blood sugar. Like carbohydrates, it has 4 calories per gram. And like both, you couldn't live without it.

When digested and absorbed, protein foods are broken down into amino acids. As schoolchildren, we all learned that amino acids are the body's building blocks, which is a simple way of saying they are used to make and repair every inch of the body: skin, hair, muscles, organs, and bones, as well as digestive enzymes, hormones, and the components of the immune system. Cells and even genes are made of protein, and proteins are used to repair damaged DNA. Our bodies wouldn't grow and our brains wouldn't develop without the help of protein. Protein is also a source of energy, but it is harder for the body to use protein than glucose and fat.

Protein is most abundantly available from animal sources—meat, fish, and shellfish—as well as eggs, cheese, and other dairy products. Vegetarians can get enough protein from vegetables, especially beans and bean products such as tofu and tempeh.

Shellfish is a rich source of protein and, compared to meat, much lower in fat.

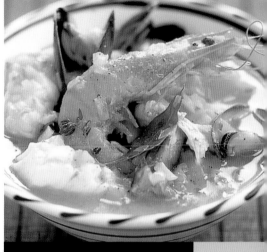

How Much Do You Need?

Most of us eat far more protein than we really need. About a half gram per pound of body weight is sufficient for an adult. So, if you weigh 150 pounds, 75 grams (less than 3 ounces) of protein will do the trick. The rest will be stored in the liver and muscles, and the overflow will be converted and stored as fat until (and unless) it is needed for energy.

Babies and children need more protein *per pound of weight* than adults, in order to support their rapid growth and development. One and a half grams per pound of body weight is recommended in the first year of life; after that, one gram per pound is needed through adolescence.

Where Protein Comes From

- Meat, including organ meat
- Fish
- Shellfish
- Eggs
- Cheese
- Milk products, including yogurt and cottage cheese
- Dried beans and legumes
- Cereal grains
- Nuts and nut butters
- Seeds and seed pastes

Where It Goes

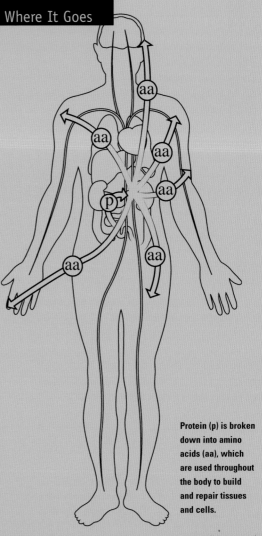

Protein (p) is broken down into amino acids (aa), which are used throughout the body to build and repair tissues and cells.

The *gi* Handbook

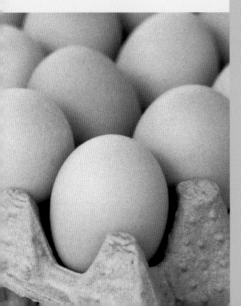

Why the G.I. Matters

The G.I. measures not what or how much is *in* food, but how quickly the body *processes* each component of the food you eat. The rate and amount of glucose entering the bloodstream has a profound effect on the normal operation of the body. Too much too soon and too fast can be extremely damaging. It not only makes the body store fat more readily and withdraw it from storage less easily, it also taxes the effectiveness and supply of insulin.

What the Experts Say

Understanding and making food choices according to the G.I. is a scientifically based way of working with the normal processes of the body to prevent weight gain, foster weight loss, and slow or halt the development of severe health problems ranging from Type 2 diabetes to cardiovascular disease.

Studies of diets based on the G.I. found that foods in the lower range aided weight reduction, as well as the management of Type 2 diabetes. People on low-G.I. diets were less likely to overeat since they felt fuller longer. It is believed that low-G.I. foods play a role in preserving islet cell function and therefore the normal production and secretion of insulin. Low-G.I. diets also appear to reduce levels of C-reactive protein, one of the major inflammatory factors associated with the development of coronary heart disease, and to have a beneficial effect on cholesterol levels, in particular by raising HDL.

G.I. and Your Body

Low-G.I. foods are converted to glucose slowly and gradually.

▶ Insulin secretion is equally slow and gradual.

▶ Insulin potency and supply are preserved.

▶ Fat storage and retrieval follow a normal pattern based on energy requirements.

Low-G.I. foods also:

▶ Raise HDL, the "good" cholesterol.

▶ Reduce C-reactive protein, an inflammatory factor.

High-G.I. foods raise the level of glucose in the blood quickly and dramatically.

▶ In response, islet cells of the pancreas release large amounts of insulin to clear the glucose.

▶ Over time, insulin become less effective at clearing glucose (glucose resistance) and the islet cells make less of it (insulin exhaustion).

▶ Insulin helps the body convert glucose for fat storage.

▶ Insulin makes it harder for the body to withdraw fat for energy.

The G.I. Is a Work in Progress

The first G.I. list, which accompanied Dr. Jenkins' paper introducing the G.I. in the *American Journal of Clinical Nutrition* in 1981, contained 51 foods. In 1995, an article in that same journal expanded the list to 250 foods, following up with a longer list in 2002. Even so, of all the hundreds of thousands of individual foods and food combinations, fewer than 1,000 have undergone G.I. testing.

This is in contrast to calorie count and nutrient content, which are contained in a vast nutrient database that is maintained by the U.S. Department of Agriculture (USDA), with data drawn from numerous sources, including from food manufacturers. G.I. testing, a long and complicated process, is done in only a few laboratories in the world. Moreover, individual foods are tested, not whole meals—the way most of us eat—so there is no information on how other carbohydrate and non-carbohydrate foods might influence the rate of digestion. Finally, unlike calories (which are an objective measure of the amount of heat energy a food contains), and fat, protein, and carbohydrate (other objective measures of *what* a food contains), G.I. refers to *how* the body uses that food. Every body is different: young or old, healthy or ill, active or sedentary, muscular or slight, overweight or underweight, male or female.

Research on the glycemic effect of food combinations is ongoing. Over time, more foods will be tested, and it is even possible that one day packaged foods will be labeled to indicate their G.I. Whether that is a good thing remains to be seen. It may help people make wiser food choices or it may sow more confusion, encouraging consumers to keep track of yet more numbers while they try to hear the health message amid the babble of the food industry.

Still, the glycemic index does help us to identify "good" and "bad" carbs and makes it possible for us to eat a balanced diet without succumbing to indiscriminate "carbophobia." It can be used as a meal-planning tool by people with diabetes or prediabetic conditions. It also makes sense as a cornerstone of a successful weight-loss strategy. More than anything else, it encourages a way of eating that can be followed throughout a lifetime, because it does not outlaw a whole class of foods, does not require obsessive number crunching, but does provide a wide range of choices from among the most satisfying foods.

The G.I. is the key to a whole new way of thinking about food. It is a lifelong approach to eating that will help you and your loved ones get healthy and stay that way.

Summing Up: What Is the Glycemic Index?

▶ The G.I. classifies carbohydrates according to how they affect blood sugar levels.

▶ High-G.I. foods are digested quickly and cause spikes in blood sugar. Low-G.I. foods are digested slowly, keeping blood sugar levels low and steady.

▶ A slow and gradual rise in blood sugar preserves the strength and supply of insulin, the master hormone of metabolism.

▶ The G.I. includes carbohydrates only.

▶ Carbohydrates are a large group of nutrients ranging from simple sugars to more complex starches and highly complex fiber.

▶ Carbohydrates are broken down into glucose, a simple sugar, in the course of digestion.

▶ Refined grains and flours, potatoes, sugar and other sweeteners are high-G.I. carbohydrates.

▶ Carbohydrates are essential to life and health. A diet that forbids or severely restricts carbohydrate intake is not a healthy diet.

▶ The best sources of low-G.I. carbohydrates are fresh fruits, non-starchy vegetables, dried beans and legumes, and whole grains.

▶ Although it is a carbohydrate, fiber is a "no-G.I., no-calorie" bonus. Eat 25–30 grams a day.

▶ Calories count. If you take in more than you use, you will gain weight.

▶ The G.I. is an essential tool for making healthy food choices.

▶ Combined with exercise, calorie intake that matches energy needs, and not smoking, the G.I. will help you live a long and healthy life.

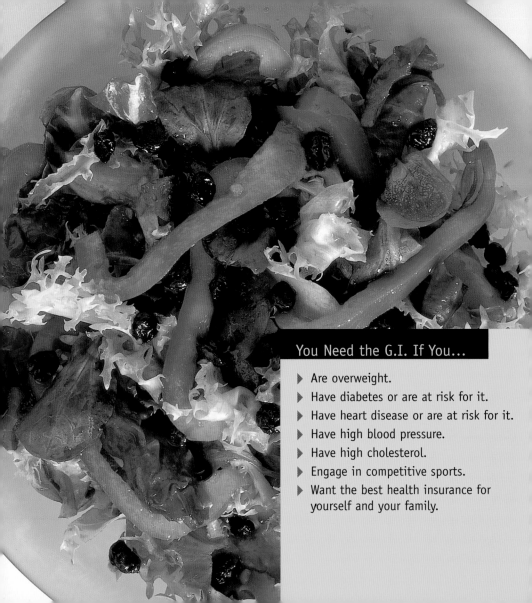

You Need the G.I. If You...

▶ Are overweight.
▶ Have diabetes or are at risk for it.
▶ Have heart disease or are at risk for it.
▶ Have high blood pressure.
▶ Have high cholesterol.
▶ Engage in competitive sports.
▶ Want the best health insurance for yourself and your family.

2 Who Needs the Glycemic Index?

Anybody who wants to be healthy and stay that way! Being aware of the G.I. content of the food you eat will help you to make wise food choices and maintain a normal weight. Eating low-G.I. foods will also help you lose weight if you need to.

Who Can Benefit?

If you are overweight, you have a greatly increased risk of developing Type 2 diabetes. Modifying your diet is among the most important strategies for avoiding the onset of this disabling and potentially deadly disease, and the G.I. is the ultimate weapon in the battle.

If you already have diabetes, you know that tightly controlling your blood sugar level throughout the day and night is essential. The G.I. is your basic tool for keeping your blood sugar in check.

If you or close family members have heart disease, high blood pressure, or a history of strokes, many health-care professionals believe you can reduce the risks to yourself by using the G.I. as a guide to what you eat.

If you engage in competitive sports or regularly pursue any other type of activity that makes large demands on your energy, being G.I.-aware can help ensure you have the fuel you need to keep going.

If you want to live a long and healthy life, choosing foods according to the G.I. is the keystone of an effective preventive health strategy.

The G.I. is not a diet. It is a way of working with your metabolism to get what you need out of the food you eat without putting your health at risk.

Life is more than just a bowl of salad when the G.I. guides your food choices. Here's to a long life and a healthier you!

Overweight and At Risk

Recently, the U.S. federal Department of Health and Human Services (HHS) officially branded obesity an illness.

In the words of HHS Secretary Tommy Thompson, "Obesity is a critical public health problem in our country that causes millions of Americans to suffer unnecessary health problems and to die prematurely."

The Gruesome Threesome

Obesity, Type 2 diabetes, and cardiovascular disease may seem like three separate health problems. The truth is, there is a cause and effect relationship among the three. People who are overweight are at extremely high risk for Type 2 diabetes. The metabolic disturbances that characterize diabetes contribute to obesity and make weight loss more difficult by enhancing fat storage, especially in the abdominal

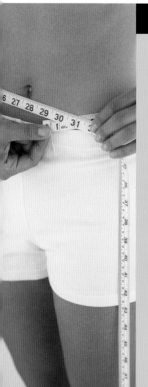

Health Risks Associated with Being Overweight

▶ Cardiovascular diseases, including: Atherosclerosis (clogged arteries), atrial fibrillation (irregular heartbeat), coronary artery disease, hypertension (high blood pressure)

▶ Type 2 diabetes

▶ Gall bladder disease and gallstones

▶ Heart attack

▶ High cholesterol

Your weight and waistline are not about vanity. They're matters of life and death.

▶ Lung and other breathing problems, including: Asthma, shortness of breath, sleep apnea (periods of interrupted breathing while asleep)

▶ Pain, including: Arthritis, back pain, gout, joint pain

▶ Stroke

In addition, it has been suggested that people who are overweight have a higher incidence of some cancers, including breast, uterine, prostate, and colon cancers.

area. This "apple" body shape is called central obesity and it is a major risk factor for heart attack. Heart and circulatory problems (cardiovascular disease) go hand in hand with Type 2 diabetes and often warn of its development.

In fact, many heart and circulatory problems show up as much as a decade before the symptoms of Type 2 diabetes are recognizable and the disease is finally diagnosed.

Are You Overweight?

In the U.S., the National Institutes of Health defines being overweight in terms of body mass index, or B.M.I., a formula that takes into account both height and weight. According to the NIH guidelines, a B.M.I. of over 25 is considered overweight and a B.M.I. of 30 or more is considered obese. *Morbid obesity* is being so severely overweight (B.M.I. of 40 or more) as to limit normal activities, disturb normal body functions, and cause disease.

You can find your B.M.I. by using the chart on page 56. All you need to know is your height and weight. First, start by finding your height in the left-hand column. Then move to the right until you reach your weight. Look at the top of that column to establish your B.M.I.

Metabolic Syndrome

Remember metabolic syndrome, also known as Syndrome X (*see page 25*), the group of disorders linked to Type 2 diabetes, heart disease, and stroke? Well, X marks the spot where obesity, high cholesterol, high blood pressure, and insulin defects come together. Rates of metabolic syndrome more than doubled in the last decade of the twentieth century. During that period, more Americans tipped the scales into obesity. No one doubts the connection.

B.M.I. = Body Mass Index

The body mass index has replaced the old familiar weight tables that tell us if our weight is above or below normal or just where it ought to be.

A B.M.I. of:	Is considered:
Less than 18	Underweight
18–24	Desirable weight
25–29	Overweight
30–40	Obese
More than 40	Severely obese

To use the table below, find your height in the left-hand column labeled "Height." Then move across until you reach your weight (in pounds, rounded off). The number at the top of that column is your B.M.I. Then look on page 55 to see whether your weight is in the desirable range.

BMI	19	20	21	22	23	24	25	26	27	28	29	30	31	32	33	34	35
Height (inches)							Body weight (pounds)										
58	91	96	100	105	110	115	119	124	129	134	138	143	148	153	158	162	167
59	94	99	104	109	114	119	124	128	133	138	143	148	153	158	163	168	173
60	97	102	107	112	118	123	128	133	138	143	148	153	158	163	168	174	179
61	100	106	11	116	122	122	127	132	137	143	148	153	164	169	174	180	185
62	104	109	115	120	126	131	136	142	147	153	158	164	169	175	180	186	191
63	107	113	118	124	130	135	141	146	152	158	163	169	175	180	186	191	197
64	110	116	122	128	134	140	145	151	157	163	169	174	180	186	192	197	204
65	114	120	126	132	138	144	150	156	162	168	174	180	186	192	198	204	210
66	118	124	130	136	142	148	155	161	167	173	179	186	192	198	204	210	216
67	121	127	134	140	146	153	159	166	172	178	185	191	198	204	211	217	223
68	125	131	138	144	151	158	164	171	177	184	190	197	203	210	216	223	230
69	128	135	142	149	155	162	168	176	182	189	196	203	209	216	223	230	236
70	132	139	146	153	160	167	174	181	188	195	202	209	216	222	229	236	243
71	136	143	150	157	165	172	179	186	193	200	208	215	222	229	236	243	250
72	140	147	154	162	169	177	184	191	199	206	213	221	228	235	242	250	258
73	144	151	159	166	174	182	189	197	204	212	219	227	235	242	250	257	265
74	148	155	163	171	179	186	194	202	210	218	225	233	241	249	256	264	272
75	152	160	168	176	184	192	200	208	216	224	232	240	248	256	264	272	279
76	156	164	172	180	189	197	205	213	221	230	238	246	254	263	271	279	287

How the G.I. Can Help You Lose Weight

The dramatic rise in obesity seen in the past decade has been tied to recommendations that we eat less fat. The catch is that we need to replace that fat with something. It can't be replaced with protein because most protein foods are also relatively high in fat, so we turned to carbohydrates—with the blessing of the USDA and its tipsy food pyramid. Carb consumption went way up as we packed in starchy and sugary foods, convinced we were fending off weight and other health problems. Many public health experts see that as an explanation for the failure of the public to lose weight, even when cutting fat.

When low-fat/high-carb diets did not work, there was a backlash that continues to reverberate in the weight-loss world. Suddenly carbs were bad, fat okay, and calories irrelevant. This way of thinking is as misguided as saying that any kind of carbs is better than any kind of fat. The truth, as you now know, lies in the fact that different kinds of carbohydrates affect blood sugar and insulin levels in different ways. Sudden highs result in fat conservation.

The G.I. offers a new way of looking at the good advice to reduce harmful fats without substituting the wrong carbohydrates. It tells you which carbohydrate foods cause blood sugar to seesaw and which keep it low and steady. That, in turn, avoids spikes in insulin secretion and disturbances of fat storage that result.

Should you or shouldn't you? The G.I. helps you answer that question.

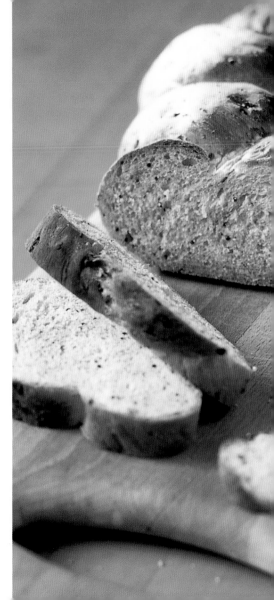

Who Needs the Glycemic Index?

Diabetes Numbers

Percentage of diabetes incidence in people over 20, by age group, in the United States. Among children and adolescents, the incidence is 0.25%.

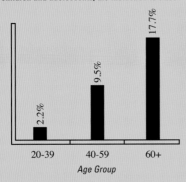

Age Group

Total incidence of diabetes (in millions) for adults, in the United States.

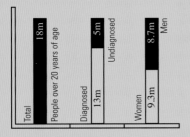

Source: National Health Interview Survey, 1999–2001, and National Health Examination Survey, 1999–2000

A Diabetes Epidemic

"Increasing intakes of refined carbohydrate (corn syrup) concomitant with decreasing intakes of fiber paralleled the upward trend in the prevalence of Type 2 diabetes observed in the United States during the 20th Century." That's the bad news according to an "ecologic assessment" that was published in the *American Journal of Clinical Nutrition* in 2004, which linked the increased consumption of refined carbohydrates to what public health experts call an epidemic of diabetes.

What Is Diabetes?

Diabetes is a group of metabolic disorders in which abnormally high blood sugar levels cause widespread damage, including impaired circulation and healing ability, susceptibility to infection, kidney failure, and blindness. The two most common forms are Type 1 and Type 2. In both, the problem is insulin.

At least 18 million Americans —6.3% of the total population —have diabetes, but more than one-third do not know it.

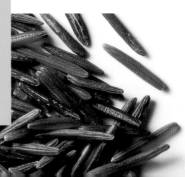

Insulin

Remember insulin, the master hormone? Insulin plays a role in many different functions and acts on many different organs and tissues in the human body. It governs how the body treats glucose—specifically, how, when, and where it is stored and withdrawn for use as a fuel source.

Levels of insulin rise in response and in proportion to the presence of glucose in the blood when carbohydrates are eaten; they subside when the insulin has done its work. Foods that result in high insulin secretion cause the body to store fat; foods that keep glucose—and, therefore, insulin—at lower levels cause the body to burn fat rather than storing it.

Insulin abnormalities are seen in both diabetes and obesity. They are also associated with inflammation and disordered blood coagulation that contribute to cardiovascular disease, especially heart attacks and strokes.

Diabetes: What Type?

Type 1 diabetes is an autoimmune disease in which the islet cells of the pancreas are damaged and do not produce any insulin. Because it usually develops before the age of 20, it has also been called *juvenile diabetes*. There is no cure, so young people with Type 1 grow up to be adults with Type 1, and they need injected insulin throughout their lives.

Type 2 diabetes is a progressive disease that is linked to obesity, a sedentary lifestyle, and heredity. Over time, insulin becomes less effective at clearing glucose from the blood. This is termed insulin resistance. The islet cells of the pancreas respond by making more insulin, which becomes increasingly ineffective. Eventually, the islet cells are exhausted and stop producing insulin. Total insulin exhaustion may be delayed by changes in diet, weight loss, and regular exercise. Many people also have to take medicines to control their blood sugar, and eventually will need insulin injections. Because obesity and Type 2 diabetes are related, both as cause and effect, people who are newly diagnosed with the disease are urged to get their B.M.I. below 25 and keep it there.

Tight Control Is the Key

Diabetes cannot be cured; it can only be managed, with drugs, insulin, or both. In addition, blood sugar levels must be closely monitored to avoid disabling and life-threatening complications. People with diabetes must prick a fingertip and test a small drop of blood many times a day to ensure that their glucose level remains low and steady, with no sharp peaks or deep valleys. In addition, they must pay strict attention to every morsel of food they eat.

Tight control has revolutionized diabetes management, but it is a lot of work for the person with diabetes. Choosing foods with an awareness of their glycemic index can make the task easier. It can also help with the weight loss that is the first thing physicians will prescribe after diagnosing Type 2 diabetes. If you have diabetes of either type, talk to your doctor or your diabetes educator about how you can best incorporate the G.I. into your meal and weight-loss planning.

Diabetes Complications

The complications of diabetes are numerous and serious, affecting many body systems and often acting in a vicious cycle that feeds upon itself. Among them are:

▶ Nerve damage, leading to pain and numbness

▶ Impaired circulation, leading to:
  Eye damage, which may lead to blindness

▶ Low resistance to infection, which leads to:
  Slow healing of wounds, which may lead to further infection

▶ Gangrene, typically in the toes, feet, and lower legs, leading to amputation

▶ Ketoacidosis, which may lead to coma and death

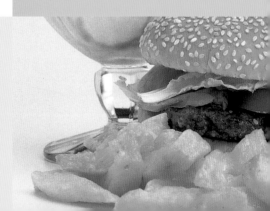

Children who subsist on burgers and fries develop weight-related health problems usually seen only in adults.

It's *Not* Juvenile Diabetes

Young people may have it, but it's not juvenile (Type 1) diabetes. They are not suffering from an autoimmune disease with no apparent cause that cannot be avoided with lifestyle changes. This is Type 2 and it can be delayed, if not prevented. But it means starting now to help children make the changes that will make a difference.

It is absolutely essential that kids stop gorging themselves on sugary, greasy, starchy junk foods and start getting much more exercise. The effort begins at home, but it has to extend to the schools and other institutions that influence what our children eat and what they do with their free time.

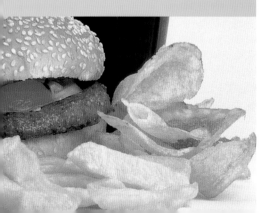

Children at Risk

Type 2 diabetes used to be considered a disorder of adulthood, usually middle age. It is still true that most people with the disease are over 60, but there has been an alarming increase in the number of young people diagnosed with prediabetic conditions and full-blown diabetes itself. The same risk factors apply: heredity, being overweight, and a sedentary lifestyle. Nothing can be done about hereditary factors, but the blame for the early onset of Type 2 diabetes can be laid squarely on the dramatic increase in obesity among the young and the distressing decrease in the amount of physical activity in this same age group. No small part of that blame starts at the door of fast food restaurants, those magnets for children, busy families, and people on the go. They sell meals that are quick, easy, and relatively cheap, but they are combat zones for anyone who is trying to raise healthy children with good eating habits.

More and more parents are hearing from pediatricians that their children and teens are seriously overweight and have high blood pressure, abnormal cholesterol and triglyceride levels, and signs of insulin resistance. What this means is that young people are entering adulthood with a head start on the severe health problems that have previously not been seen until middle age. It adds up to an extra 20 or more years of abnormal cholesterol and high blood pressure, and of defects in insulin secretion—time enough to develop the heart, circulatory, and metabolic problems that cripple and kill.

Kids Count

Study after study shows that American kids are eating more high-G.I. foods than they used to: candy and other sweets, soft drinks, junk food, fast food, sweetened cereals made from processed grains, and lots and lots of high fructose corn syrup. A little label reading will tell you how deeply corn syrup has invaded our food supply. You'll find it even in foods that do not taste particularly sweet, such as peanut butter, ketchup, bottled salad dressings, and just about every product on the snack food shelves. Not only are children eating more junk, they are eating less of what they should be eating: fresh fruits and vegetables, whole grains, and dairy products (that is, low-fat milk, yogurt, and cheese, not ice cream). Not only are they gaining weight, they are experiencing spikes in blood sugar many times a day, after every carb-laden meal and snack, setting them up for insulin resistance, insulin exhaustion, and Type 2 diabetes.

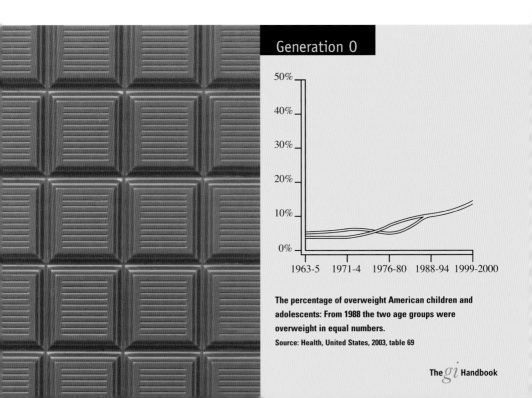

Generation 0

The percentage of overweight American children and adolescents: From 1988 the two age groups were overweight in equal numbers.
Source: Health, United States, 2003, table 69

Couch Potatoes and Other Bad Carbs

Team sports, recreational activities, homework, music lessons and other extracurricular activities, television, video games, computer time—there are only so many hours in the day. Something has got to give and it's clear that physical activity has gotten the boot. Schools, which ought to be preaching *and* practicing physical fitness and good nutrition, have cut back on gym classes and team sports, citing the need to allocate limited time and funds to academic subjects. At the same time, many schools have invited soft drink companies to install soda and snack machines in school buildings. So they have essentially traded physical activity for high fructose corn syrup as a way of making ends meet, and an entire generation will end up footing the bill.

Parents who care about their children's health should raise their voices in protest and work with local schools to reverse this unhealthy trend. It has worked in some communities. Try it in yours.

By the beginning of the twenty-first century, 15 percent of American children were overweight compared to only 5 percent in 1970. That same period saw a dramatic decline in physical activity among the young: During the 1970s, 80 percent engaged in some kind of organized physical activity every day, compared to only 20 percent of children today.

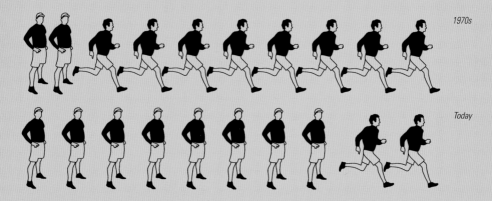

1970s

Today

Give Them a Healthy Start

These are the facts:

▶ Overweight children grow up to become overweight adults.

▶ Children with one or more overweight parents are more likely to be overweight than are children with two parents whose weight is normal.

▶ Children who develop a taste for sweets and starchy junk food enter adulthood with unhealthy eating habits that are hard to break.

What Can Parents Do to Start Children Out on the Right Path?

If your child is overweight, inactive, or both, work with your pediatrician to devise an eating and exercise plan that will slow weight gain as your child grows.

Do not try to put your child on a weight-loss diet unless the doctor advises it.

Do get your entire family involved in fun activities—ranging from an after-dinner walk or a game of catch to weekend bike rides and active summer vacations. Other ideas to try out include dog walking, indoor and outdoor chores, and after-school sports.

What Parents Can Do

▶ Include at least 30 minutes of activity in every day, for both you and your children.

▶ Restrict children's intake of sweet soft drinks and noncitrus juices.

▶ Add whole grains, nonstarchy vegetables, and fresh fruit to meals throughout the day.

▶ Fill the refrigerator and pantry with low- to medium-G.I. snacks and beverages.

▶ Don't buy sugary, salty, greasy snack foods and don't allow them in your house.

▶ Send your kids off to school with their tummies full of a nutritious low- to medium-G.I. breakfast and a homemade lunch that will keep their brains and bodies nourished.

▶ Be a good role model by achieving and maintaining normal weight and eating a healthy, balanced diet.

▶ Raise your voice and use your influence to get daily physical education back in school and vending machines out!

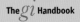

If your child is home alone after school with no one to discourage sedentary pastimes, make a deal. For every half hour in front of the television or computer screen, ask your child to commit to a half hour in motion. It can be as simple as putting on some music and dancing around the room or playing a game of tag in the backyard. If your child has tons of homework, suggest ten minutes of stretching for every hour of studying. Make a game of it, using a kitchen timer or stopwatch and tokens or coupons that you make together to barter "sitting down" time for "get up and go" time.

Give your kids a running start. Habits that begin in childhood are difficult to break—even the healthy ones!

It is especially important for parents to use their influence when their children are at home and developing their tastes and eating habits. Once they leave the nest, young people tend to gain additional weight. The "freshman 15" is a well-known phenomenon among new college students, who typically gain about 15 pounds in their first year of eating away from home. The villains seem to be irregular meals, especially fast food and snacks that are high in sugar and trans fats, combined with more stress and less exercise.

Health-wise parents send their kids off to college with a strong nutritional foundation so that they do not enter adulthood overweight and with poor eating habits.

A G.I. Bill for the Golden Years

Like childhood, old age is a time of physical change. Decreased hormones mean muscle mass and fat deposits shrink, bones become more fragile, skin and blood vessels more delicate, balance and vision less reliable. As a result, older people tend to be less active and their health often declines. For some, this may lead to weight gain and, even if they were previously healthy, diabetes and heart problems that may have been brewing undetected for years.

Even if they have been advised to lose weight or change their eating patterns for other health reasons, seniors especially should not go on one-dimensional diets or any diet that alters the metabolism, is deficient in vitamins and minerals, changes their bowel habits, unbalances their electrolytes (an essential aspect of body chemistry), causes mineral loss from bones, or draws on muscle stores of glycogen. Instead, they should choose foods that will help them lose, gain, or maintain weight, as needed; avoid constipation; and preserve muscle and bone mass and a healthy fat cushion while keeping blood sugar, cholesterol levels, and blood pressure in check.

Sound like a tall order? It isn't when the G.I. is the guide. A balanced diet that emphasizes low-G.I. carbohydrates, fiber, unsaturated fats, and sufficient protein is the best prescription for healthy aging.

The importance of good nutrition increases as we grow older. Hearty soups are rich sources of nutrients and easy to prepare and eat.

Here's to Healthy Aging

▶ Stay active, both physically and mentally.

▶ Maintain your normal weight.

▶ Eat a balanced diet rich in low-G.I. foods and fiber and low in starchy and sugary foods and saturated fat.

▶ Get vital vitamins and minerals from whole grains, fresh fruits, and non-starchy vegetables.

▶ If you have heart and circulatory problems, high blood pressure, high cholesterol, or diabetes, follow your doctor's orders and use the G.I. to guide food choices.

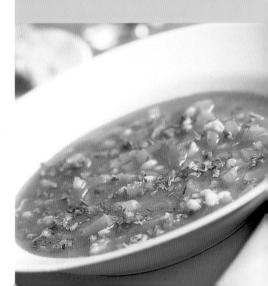

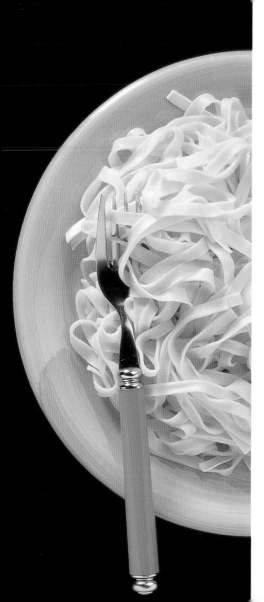

Fuel That Activity

If you exercise regularly, at the gym or with a morning jog several times a week, ride a bike on weekends, or engage in recreational sports, you are doing your heart, bones, and waistline a big favor, but you do not need to eat like a professional athlete. If, however, you are a body builder, a competitive athlete, or have a job that requires high-energy expenditure, endurance, and strength, turning the G.I. on its head, so to speak, can work for you.

Why Athletes Need Extra Carbs

Athletes digest carbohydrates just like the rest of us, but they have different carbohydrate needs. For starters, they need more of them, since carbohydrates are the most readily available source of energy.

Before competition, they need to take in a large amount of low-G.I. carbs to provide a steady supply of glucose to fuel their body throughout a period of high-level exertion. That's why marathoners down huge plates of pasta, which, despite what you may have heard, is a low-G.I. carb. This pre-race "carb loading" is equivalent to gassing up before the Indy 500. *After* the event, the glucose supply is depleted and, in all likelihood, glycogen stores in the liver and muscles have also been drained. That's when they need a high-G.I. meal to help restore what they have lost.

The G.I. ensures that competitive athletes get the carbs they need when they need them.

Prevention Is More than Half the Battle

The "gruesome threesome" kills more Americans than any other illness. Happily, there is a way to fight back. Lifestyle changes can greatly reduce the risk of falling prey to one or more of these life-threatening conditions.

What the Experts Say

There is no question that the high-carb diet most Americans eat leads to elevated postprandial blood sugar, which is a risk factor for heart disease and Type 2 diabetes. Refined starches and sugar have been shown to increase insulin resistance. In addition, high-G.I. carbohydrates raise triglycerides and lower HDL, increasing the risk of cardiovascular disease. Ongoing research is seeking to uncover the reasons, but prime suspects include such technical-sounding mechanisms as oxidative stress, inflammatory factors, protein glycation, and LDL oxidation. In simple terms, a broad range of metabolic activities gone wrong contribute to the conditions that narrow blood vessels and put undue stress on the heart.

Low-G.I. carbohydrates, on the other hand, have been shown to lower triglycerides and LDL, raise HDL, and preserve insulin sensitivity, thereby lowering the risk of cardiovascular disease and metabolic syndrome. Increasing intake of unsaturated fats and fiber, the ultimate "no-G.I." carb, also reduces the likelihood of developing the syndrome. Studies of people with diabetes have shown that a low-G.I. diet improves blood sugar control.

When it comes to overweight children and teens, studies have found that coupling low-G.I. foods with reduced calories has resulted in greater weight loss than diets that emphasize reducing fat. Moreover, a low-G.I. diet is easy for kids to follow and parents to understand. When served high-G.I. meals, on the other hand, children eat more and feel less sated, a vicious cycle that leads to snacking and overeating.

People with diabetes and heart disease, and those at risk for these conditions, should aim for even lower cholesterol and blood pressure. Medication coupled with changes in diet and exercise will likely be needed to get the numbers down.

Keeping It All in Check

- ☑ B.M.I. between 18 and 24
- ☑ Waist smaller than 35 inches (women), 40 inches (men)
- ☑ LDL under 100
- ☑ HDL 60 or above
- ☑ Total cholesterol under 200
- ☑ Triglycerides under 150
- ☑ Blood pressure 120/80 or lower
- ☑ Blood sugar tested normal within the past year
- ☑ Minimum of 30 minutes of moderate activity five days a week
- ☑ Diet that emphasizes whole grains, fresh fruit, nonstarchy vegetables, and unsaturated fat
- ☑ No smoking

Summing Up: Who Needs the Glycemic Index?

▶ Many severe health problems are associated with or caused by repeated spikes in blood sugar, including obesity, insulin resistance, Type 2 diabetes, and cardiovascular disease.

▶ Making food choices from the lower range of the G.I. can prevent weight gain, help you lose weight, and prevent or slow the development of insulin resistance, Type 2 diabetes, and cardiovascular disease.

▶ People with diabetes can use the G.I. to help control blood sugar levels and maintain a healthy weight.

▶ People with heart disease or high blood pressure can use the G.I. to help manage these conditions.

▶ People who have high cholesterol and triglycerides can use the G.I. to help lower them.

▶ Parents can use the G.I. to help their children develop eating habits that will keep them healthy as they grow.

▶ Children who are overweight can use the G.I. to put them on the road to better eating.

▶ Older people can use the G.I. to help maintain a healthy weight while ensuring their nutritional needs are met.

▶ Athletes and other extremely active people can use the G.I. to ensure they get the fuel they need when they need it.

▶ People who want to stay healthy can use the G.I. to lower their risk for many chronic and potentially life-threatening diseases.

▶ The G.I. is for anyone and everyone—healthy or otherwise—who wants to make wise food choices.

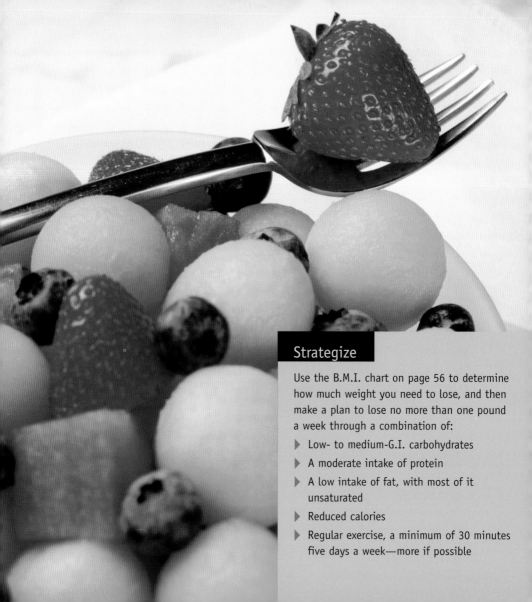

Strategize

Use the B.M.I. chart on page 56 to determine how much weight you need to lose, and then make a plan to lose no more than one pound a week through a combination of:

▶ Low- to medium-G.I. carbohydrates

▶ A moderate intake of protein

▶ A low intake of fat, with most of it unsaturated

▶ Reduced calories

▶ Regular exercise, a minimum of 30 minutes five days a week—more if possible

3 How to Use This Book

Once you understand the principles of the glycemic index and how it fits into a healthy diet, you will be able to plan meals at home and make wise selections at restaurants and social gatherings with the help of the tips and ideas in this book, and the food tables in Chapter 6.

Theory and Practice

The glycemic index rests on a sound scientific foundation that has been tested in both the laboratory and the clinic. Currently, however, the database of carbohydrate-containing foods is limited, largely because of the complexities of the testing process.

The G.I. began as a tool for researchers trying to understand more about how the body metabolizes carbohydrates and stores fat, in both sickness and health. In many ways, it remains so. Theory is one thing, but how do ordinary people put it into practice? How can the G.I. be used in the real world? The answer is: lots of ways, depending on your needs and goals.

If You Want to Lose Weight

The G.I. works with, rather than against, your metabolism to burn calories in a normal way. It helps you prevent the spikes in blood sugar and insulin that cause you to store rather than burn fat, which torpedoes so many efforts to lose weight. It offers a way of eating you can stick with: easy to follow, not overly restrictive, with a wide range of choices. It allows you to eat foods that promote "fullness" at the same time that it discourages overeating at mealtimes and keeps you from getting hungry between meals.

Fresh fruit salad is a low-G.I. treat, but check the food lists in Chapter 6 for one high-G.I. ingredient. (Here's a hint: It's the watermelon.)

If You're Just Starting Out

This book introduces you to the concept of the G.I. and helps you to make the most of your weight-loss strategies, rather than unwittingly undermining them. This is a lifelong eating plan, not a diet, so you don't have to worry about counting points and grams or keeping track of stages and phases.

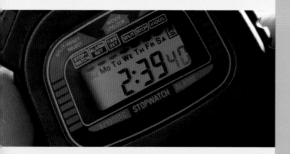

If You're in Training

The G.I. can be an important tool for athletes and other seriously active people. The finer details of when and what they need depend on the nature of the activity—its duration and whether it is stamina or strength that is most important. Body builders, for example, have a unique set of needs—in addition to bulking up, they also want to burn away fat to better define their musculature.

If you are a competitive athlete, discuss the G.I. with your trainer so that you can work together to devise an eating plan that is tailored to the specifics of your training, competition, and recovery. That way, you will be able to ensure that you have the fuel you need when you need it.

Analyze Your Eating Habits

Spend a week just observing your eating habits before you begin. Pay particular attention to:

▶ How many meals you eat in a normal day

▶ When you feel hungry

▶ What, besides hunger, triggers you to eat

▶ What foods you crave

▶ How well balanced your meals are: Are you getting enough carbohydrates? What kind of carbs are they?

You may find it helpful to keep a food journal (*see pages 112–113*).

Serious athletes can use the full range of the G.I.—low to high—while training, during competition, and in the important recovery phase that follows.

Assemble a Carb Catalog

Make a list of the carbohydrate foods you eat (column A) and the ones you avoid (column B). Look them up in the food lists in Chapter 6 (*see pages 137–165*), marking each as high, medium, and low.

Are any in the wrong column? Can you in fact eat some of the foods that you've been craving but avoiding? Should you limit or eliminate some of the foods that you've been eating?

Snack Central

▶ Ask your kids to make a list of their favorite snacks.

▶ Look the foods up together in the food lists in Chapter 6 and mark them as low, medium, or high G.I.

▶ Try to find lower G.I. trade-offs for the high-G.I. snacks.

▶ Make a deal to substitute one or two each week.

If You're Already Cutting Carbs

Whether you are watching the carbohydrate content of your meals as part of a formal diet or just on your own, this book will help you make the most of your efforts by clarifying which carbs to cut, which to eat, and why. Using the G.I. will make it possible for you to get the many benefits of carbs, as well as avoid substituting other foods that lack the benefits or add to your caloric intake. The G.I. works with any of the carb-conscious diets—indeed, it is the theoretical basis of all of them.

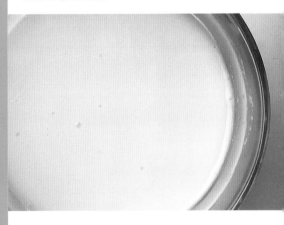

If You're Cooking for Kids

Use this book to plan family meals and build your shopping list with greater awareness of the G.I. It's the best way to ensure that your children grow up with healthy eating habits. Getting your kids involved in the planning will make it easier for them to buy into any changes that should be made.

If You're Under Doctor's Orders

No one who has medical problems that are being managed by one or more healthcare providers should make changes in diet, exercise routine, or other lifestyle factors without first discussing it with everyone involved. Ideally, one physician will be coordinating your care if you have multiple health issues, so that signals are not crossed or instructions misunderstood. A G.I.-guided eating plan can be used as an adjunct to medical care, but make sure you discuss it with your doctor first.

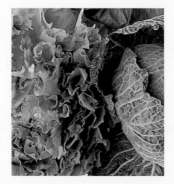

If you have diabetes, the G.I. is an important tool in meal planning. You may have also been strongly advised to lose weight. The G.I. will help you attain the goals you have set with your doctor.

If you have cholesterol problems, the G.I. will guide you to foods that help lower your LDL and raise your HDL. Cutting saturated fat and cholesterol from your diet and, in accordance with new guidelines, taking a cholesterol-lowering drug must also be part of the plan.

If you have high blood pressure, the G.I. will work in conjunction with medication and other interventions your doctor may recommend to get your blood pressure under control.

If you are a senior citizen and have multiple health problems, the G.I. can ensure you get all the nutrients you need without disturbing your metabolism or causing potentially dangerous changes to your body.

If you just want to be healthy, use the G.I. to guide your food choices and reduce your risk for metabolic syndrome and the life-threatening conditions that go along with it.

The G.I. in the Real World

The more you eat out, the less control you have over exactly what goes into your mouth. However, when 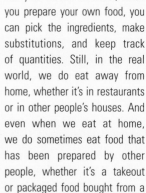 you prepare your own food, you can pick the ingredients, make substitutions, and keep track of quantities. Still, in the real world, we do eat away from home, whether it's in restaurants or in other people's houses. And even when we eat at home, we do sometimes eat food that has been prepared by other people, whether it's a takeout or packaged food bought from a supermarket. For example, when you make a pot of vegetable beef soup, you know exactly what's in it, and you can leave out the potatoes and add barley instead. But you do not have that choice if the soup comes from a can or from the hot-pot at your local deli. Canned soup at least has a label you can read, though you may not like what's on it once you start thinking in terms of the glycemic index and glycemic load (*see opposite*).

What is Glycemic Load?

Glycemic load, or G.L., is an important concept that brings the glycemic index into the real world—the world in which you eat every day. It combines the G.I. of a food with the actual amount of pure carbohydrate in a serving of that food. That is, it accurately reflects *how much* glucose will be hitting your bloodstream shortly after you swallow. The effect of glucose on insulin levels is dose-dependent. Lots of glucose needs lots of insulin to move it along out of the blood and into storage.

Although glycemic load is important for researchers, it is neither practical nor sensible for us to figure out the G.L. of everything we eat. Understanding the concept is important, however.

Glycemic index is always based on 50 grams of carbohydrate, which is a bit less than 2 ounces.

You may eat more, or perhaps even less, than that. Regardless of how much you eat, the G.I. remains the same, but the G.L. does not. For example, one teaspoon of table sugar (sucrose) has a G.I. in the middle of the medium range (about 65); so does one tablespoon.

The G.L. of that teaspoonful is about 7, whereas a tablespoonful has a G.L. of about 20. The formula for finding the G.L. is: G.I. x carbohydrate grams per serving ÷ 100 = G.L.

But should you do the math every time you think about putting food in your mouth? No. Instead, be aware of whether the carb-containing foods you eat are low, medium, or high G.I., and pay attention to the serving size. A small taste of a high-G.I. food may have the same G.L. as a triple helping of a low-G.I. food, so be honest with yourself when you make the choice between the two.

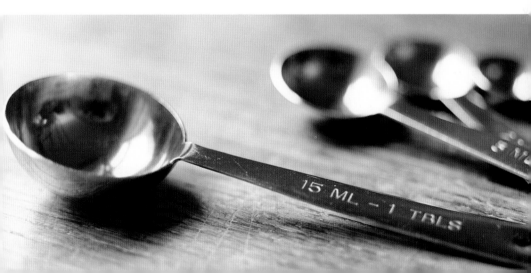

G.I.-Free Carbs

G.I. testing has not been done for foods that contain so few carbohydrates that it would take a boatload to add up to 50 grams of carbs. Celery, lettuce, and other greens are in this category. A cup of shredded romaine, for example, contains about 1.5 grams of carbohydrate, so the test subject would have to eat more than 30 cups of the stuff, *in one sitting*!

Luckily for us, that means we can have as much green salad as we like and get the benefits of the vitamins, minerals, and fiber without worrying one bit about raising our blood sugar levels. Scan the vegetable section of the food lists in Chapter 6 for more "all-you-can-eat" carbs.

At the Supermarket

Even if you cook most of what you and your family eat, the supermarket is part of your real world. These days it's also a tower of Babel, with products in every aisle crying about how low, how healthy, how smart, how low-impact their carbs are; boasting about their net carbs, not to mention that they are cholesterol-free (though they may harbor trans fats) or trans-fat free (though they may be loaded with high fructose corn syrup). Old standbys are wearing new clothes and boasting about their healthy benefits.

In simpler times, food manufacturers hoping to catch the attention of the dieting consumer had only to feature the words *low calorie* on their packages. Next came the finer distinction of *reduced calories* and *light* (or *lite*). When the focus turned to fats, *low fat*, *nonfat*, and *reduced fat* joined the chorus.

Then came the carb revolution. Suddenly we all rushed to the meat and poultry cases, deserting the staples—cereals, pastas, and the staff of life, bread. Even the old reliables in the produce department

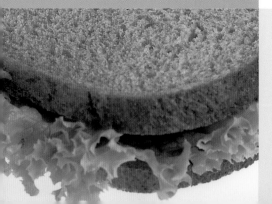

The package may say "low net carbs," but this airy whole-wheat bread is not low G.I. Dense, dark bread with visible whole grains is a better choice.

—fresh fruits and vegetables—were cast in a questionable light, with little to defend themselves, since fresh produce is not required by law to carry nutrition labels and most come unpackaged—and thus have no wrapping to advertise their health benefits.

That put food manufacturers into survival mode—tossing bran and other fibers into anything they could think of, looking for palatable sugar substitutes, and reformulating, repackaging, and retooling their marketing message. The Food and Drug Administration (FDA), the federal agency that polices food labels as well as setting nutritional guidelines, has been running to catch up, though with the speed of a lumbering hippo. It is still wrestling with the sugar question and continues to be vague about distinctions among different kinds of carbs. At present, shoppers have little to guide them in this strange new landscape. Think of this book as a map and phrasebook combined. It will help you translate the babble and navigate the shoals as you push your shopping cart in search of something healthy to eat.

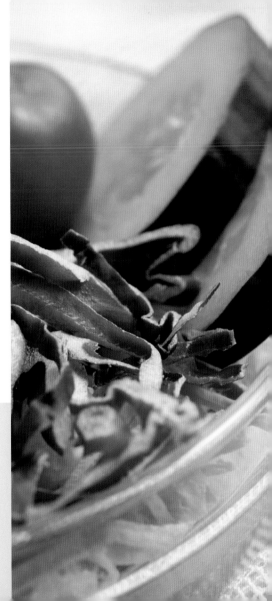

From asparagus to zucchini, most of your favorite vegetables are G.I.-free carbs—all you can eat, plus vitamins, minerals, and fiber galore!

The FDA strictly regulates what food labels can say. It is a violation to claim that something is low G.I. if it is not. But you won't actually find any mention of the glycemic index on food packaging, at least not in the U.S. Instead, you will find the words *net carbs* or some variation of this term, and often instructions on how to figure them out. Basically, grams of fiber are subtracted from total carbohydrate grams. That's fine, since fiber does not raise blood sugar. But this tells you nothing about what kind the remaining carbs are or what their G.I. is.

Net carbs *are not* the same as G.I. Remember, an extremely limited number of foods have been tested for G.I., and of those, even fewer are to be found on typical American supermarket shelves.

A Reading Lesson

The FDA governs the realm of food labeling in America. It has stipulated that one part of each food label must list ingredients in order of weight. A second part, called the Nutrition Facts panel, must contain specific information about the macro- and micronutrient content.

The smartest thing you can do for yourself and your family is to become an avid reader of food labels. Do not buy anything until you have checked what's in it. The FDA web site offers an excellent tutorial on how to read food labels (*see Useful Web Sites on pages 168–169*). For the purposes of this book, we shall focus on just a few features.

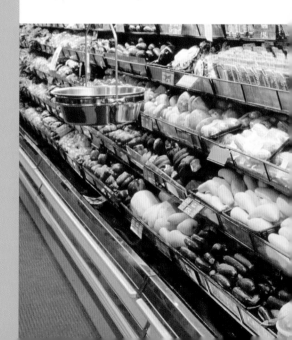

You won't find a nutrition facts label on unpackaged fresh produce. Look up the G.I. before you buy.

Serving Size: Everything that follows refers to what's in a serving, not what's in the entire package. Ignoring serving size is the biggest mistake people make, and is also the leading cause of overeating. You don't need to weigh or measure each serving if you pay attention to the next item.

Servings Per Container: If the number is more than 1, that means, "don't eat the whole thing!" In this case, half the package or container is a serving.

Trans Fat: This is very bad fat. What's left? Subtract the grams of bad and very bad fat and you're left with unsaturated fat, the good stuff.

Dietary Fiber: In this case, there's none, but if there were any, you could figure out how much starch is in the food by subtracting fiber and the next item from the total carbohydrate figure.

Calories: Remember, this is per serving, and calories do count.

Total Fat: Every gram contains nine calories. You want to keep your fat intake to no more than 30 percent of total calorie intake. Do the math.

Saturated Fat: This is bad fat.

Total Carbohydrate: Every gram has 4 calories. This does not tell you anything about the G.I.

Sugars: This can be anything from glucose and sucrose to high-fructose corn syrup or honey. Check the ingredient list to see what the sugars are (*see page 116 for a list of sugar aliases*).

Nutrition Facts

Serving Size 1 cup (228g)

Servings Per Container 2

Amount Per Serving

Calories 250   Calories from Fat 110

% Daily Value*

Total Fat 12g	**18%**
Saturated Fat 3g	**15%**
Trans Fat 1.5g	
Cholesterol 30mg	**10%**
Sodium 470mg	**20%**
Total Carbohydrate 31g	**10%**
Dietary Fiber 0g	**0%**
Sugars 5g	
Protein 5g	

Vitamin A	4%
Vitamin C	2%
Calcium	20%
Iron	4%

*Percent Daily Values are based on a 2,000 calorie diet. Your Daily Values may be higher or lower depending on your calorie needs:

	Calories:	2,000	2,500
Total Fat	Less than	65g	80g
Sat Fat	less than	20g	25g
Cholesterol	Less than	300mg	300mg
Sodium	Less than	2,400mg	2,400mg
Total Carbohydrate		300g	375g
Dietary Fiber		25g	30g

Home Cooking

Some experts think the decline in home cooking is partly to blame for the obesity epidemic. Under stress and out of time, many of us feed ourselves and our families takeout or packaged meals when we eat at home, and we also spend more time and money than we ought to eating in restaurants—whether we choose fast food, family style, or *haute cuisine*. Remember, the more you cook for yourself, the more control you have over exactly what you eat. This may require a paradigm shift in your life, but it is definitely worth trying.

Take a good, hard look at how many meals you and your family eat away from home in a typical week. Can you cut that figure in half? Start with breakfast, which is a minefield of sugar and refined carbohydrates when you eat out or take out. Trade your donuts and breakfast croissants for a bowl of whole grain cereal and fruit. You will be surprised what a difference it makes.

Brown-Bagging It

Pack your own lunch and, while you're at it, pack lunch for the rest of your household, too. It may take a bit of extra time, but it could add years to your life. Cook more than enough at dinnertime so you will have leftovers, and use them as the ingredients for low-G.I. sandwiches on whole-grain bread, refreshing salads, and comforting soups. Add fresh fruit for dessert or a mid-afternoon snack. If you don't have access to a refrigerator during your working day, keep your food cool with a bottle of frozen water and you won't need to resort to sugary soft drinks or sweetened ice tea.

Your children will appreciate the loving care that goes into this, especially if their lunches are packed in the latest cool lunch box or insulated bag. And, speaking of cool, a small brick of "blue ice" will keep their food that way until lunchtime. (Chapter 5 is full of ideas for filling that lunch box or brown bag, *see page 122*.)

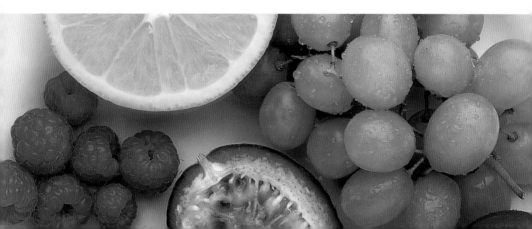

Why Rye?

Here's some good news on the sandwich front. There's no need to trade bread for a lettuce leaf wrap and deprive yourself of the myriad advantages of Lord Sandwich's great invention—portability and downright tastiness chief among them. It turns out most rye breads are low- or medium-G.I. No one is sure why, but researchers suspect it has something to do with the structure of the rye kernel. Take a look at the food lists in Chapter 6 (*see pages 137–165*) and search for rye kernel or whole grain rye and pumpernickel breads in the supermarket or health food store—the denser the slice and the more visible the grains, the better.

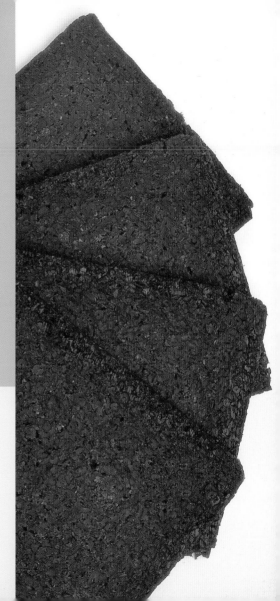

Dense rye and pumpernickel breads, with visible grains, have a lower G.I. than breads made from wheat.

Eating Out

Eating away from home is tough on dieters, no matter what diet they're on. The biggest problem isn't the ingredients; it's the out-of-control portion size. Most restaurants pile plates sky-high with far more of everything than anyone should eat.

Remember the serving size on the food label (*see page 79*)? Restaurant meals don't come with labels, so you're on your own. There are things you can do, however, to keep control of what you eat, even when you are eating out. Look at the suggested strategies given on page 83.

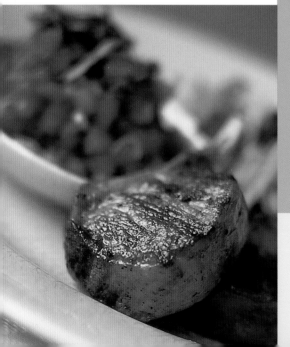

Is Pasta Passé?

Take a look at the food lists in Chapter 6 (*see pages 137–165*). The good news is that pasta is a low-G.I. food. The even better news is that whole-wheat pasta is not appreciably lower on the G.I. than the white pasta we're used to. That means that you don't have to put up with the gummy nastiness of the new "low-impact" products. Both have plenty of viscous (soluble) fiber, which slows digestion and absorption and therefore produces a low and slow rise in blood sugar.

So order that side of spaghetti primavera or toss some linguine in a pot of boiling water, cook it al dente, smother it with homemade tomato sauce, and enjoy one of your favorite comfort foods.

With a bit of care and knowledge of the G.I., you can order a restaurant meal without fear. Oversize portions are the greatest danger.

Restaurant Strategies

▶ Limit the number of meals you eat away from home as much as possible.

▶ Choose eateries with carb-conscious menus. An increasing number of establishments have them, thanks to the low-carb diet trend. If you're not sure, call ahead and ask about this.

▶ Jot down on an index card the G.I. of some of your favorite foods, especially those that you might encounter in the particular restaurant you're going to. You can slip the card out of your pocket or purse to consult while you are reading the menu.

▶ Push the bread basket out of reach and distract yourself with conversation until the food comes. If bread or rolls are served individually, smile and say: "None for me, thank you."

▶ Construct your meal with one or two appetizers, which are almost always smaller than entrées.

▶ Share your meal with one of your dining companions.

▶ Just because it's on your plate doesn't mean you have to eat it all. If it bothers you to send back a plate that isn't licked clean, ask for a "doggie bag."

▶ Dinner salads are always a safe bet, especially if you order oil and vinegar dressing and pour it on yourself.

▶ Ask for sauce and gravy on the side. That way you can spoon on a small amount or skip it all together.

▶ Substitute. Trade potatoes for an extra vegetable or a side order of pasta—yes, pasta, believe it or not.

▶ If you don't see anything on the menu you can eat, tell the server that you need a low-fat, low-starch meal, and ask what the chef can put together for you.

▶ There's no need to be secretive. Tell your dining companions about the G.I. and suggest they join you in healthy eating.

It's Easy the G.I. Way

Diets are usually about *no*, but the G.I. is full of *yes*, including some pleasant surprises. There are definitely foods you should not eat if you want to keep your blood sugar in check. But there's a lot more you *can* eat than you might imagine. As long as you keep portion size in mind and remember that calories *do* count, you will be able to enjoy a lot of delicious meals and savory snacks that won't end up on your hips and around your middle.

Striking a Balance

It's really all about balance. Although you might occasionally eat a single food—a snack consisting of just one piece of fruit, for example—most of what you eat is a combination of ingredients. How do you figure out the G.I. of everything on your plate, whether you cooked it yourself or ordered it in a restaurant?

Foods have been tested in combinations—and some complicated math has been done—to measure the glycemic response using the percentage each carbohydrate food represents of the whole meal multiplied by the G.I. of each food. But there's another wrinkle, too. The rate of digestion of carbohydrates is influenced by non-carb foods that are eaten at the same time. This seems to be especially true of fats, which slow carbohydrate digestion. This has not yet

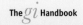

been quantified, so there is no good answer to the G.I. effect of a mixed meal.

Since you will be using G.I. ranges—high, medium, and low—rather than numbers, it is easier and certainly more practical to look at it in terms of balance rather than a mathematical calculation. For example, you may be avoiding rice because it has a high G.I. rating, but if you top it with some chili with beans and some meat and tomato sauce, and even sprinkle some grated cheddar and chopped onions on top, you will have lowered the G.I. of the entire meal. The same goes for pizza—even with a crust made from white flour. Some thin-crust pizzas qualify as low G.I. You do still have to think about calories if you are trying to lose weight, and also about cholesterol and saturated fat—especially if your cholesterol count is high. And you're not home free if you don't pay attention to portion size…

The best advice is to mostly choose foods that have low and medium G.I. ratings (or no G.I. at all), which will balance any small amount of a high G.I. food that you are really hankering for. Be aware, though, that unlike calories—which you can lend and borrow over the course of a day or even a week—the G.I. rating matters with every meal. If you eat a high G.I. meal for breakfast, a low G.I. lunch cannot undo the glycemic response.

The *gi* Handbook

Say Goodbye to Sugar?

We've been talking about sugar a lot—blood sugar, sugary snacks, high fructose corn syrup, and other hidden sugars—so the obvious conclusion is that sugar is plain bad from a glycemic point of view and you better just get used to life without it. Not so fast.

Take a look at sucrose (table sugar) in the Sweeteners section of the food lists in Chapter 6 (*see page 159*). Surprised? Yes, it's true: sucrose is a medium-G.I. carb. That means that some sugar in a low-G.I. food will not bump it into the high-G.I. range. For example, plain yogurt, yogurt with fruit and artificial sweetener, and yogurt with fruit and sugar are all comfortably in low-G.I. territory. Don't go overboard and pour on sugar with abandon, but a sprinkle here and there on food that is otherwise low-G.I. won't sink you.

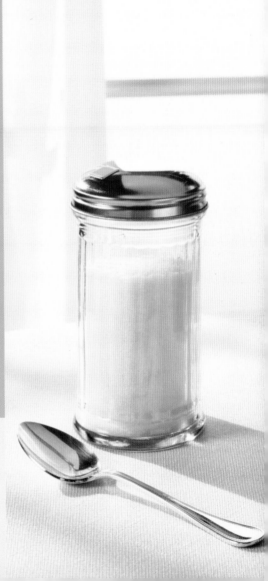

In moderation, table sugar is G.I.-safe. If you have diabetes, ask your doctor about the place of sugar in your diet.

How to Use the Food Lists

Chapter 6 contains lists of foods—fats and proteins as well as carbohydrates—to help you make wise food choices. Study the lists, looking for foods that you like. Pick out some low- and medium-G.I. foods that are unfamiliar to you and give them a try. Try to find substitutes for high-G.I. favorites among foods in the lower range. Use the lists to plan everyday meals as well as some for special occasions. You will find

that you can put together a birthday bash, a cocktail party, and even a Thanksgiving dinner with low- to medium-G.I. ingredients. Take this book along with you to the supermarket or any other place where you'll be making decisions about what to eat. It's designed to fit in your pocket or purse so it can be a ready reference whenever you need it.

Food	Serving size	Carb total (grams)	Sugar total (grams)	Fat (>5g/ serving)	G.I. rating
			17		low
Pear, raw	1 medium	25			low
• canned	½ cup	16	12		low
• in juice	½ cup	15	14		medium
• in reduced-sugar syrup	½ cup, cubed	14	13		low
Pineapple, raw	1 medium	9	5		medium
Plum, fresh, raw	1½ oz.	24	12		medium
Prunes, pitted	¼ cup	31	29		medium
Raisins	¼ cup	32	30		low
• golden (sultanas)	4 oz.	3	1		high
Strawberries, raw	1 cup, cubed	11	9		
Watermelon					none
		0	0	♥	none
Meat	3½ oz.	0	0	♥	
cooked					

Look for me in *Fats and Oils*.

Unless i extreme lean and all visi removed, a ser kind of meat h than 5 grams

We co of meat un what a 3½ looks like

added

Summing Up: How to Use This Book

▶ *The G.I. Handbook* works for everybody—individuals and families, young or old, healthy or ill, overweight or not, sedentary or extremely active.

▶ It is a real-life tool to use for planning meals and plotting out a weight-loss, preventive-health, or training strategy.

▶ It uses sound science to make sense of the newest diets.

▶ It can be used to expand your food choices while adhering to the principles of any carb-conscious diet.

▶ It is a trusty guide to help you find your way safely through the supermarket and restaurant minefields.

▶ It is full of ideas for family meals, party menus, and brown-bag lunches.

▶ It provides a yardstick for measuring carbohydrate foods in terms of their effect on your metabolism.

▶ It allows maximum flexibility in food choices, rather than banning whole groups of foods.

▶ It flags high-fat foods while it steers you to G.I.-safe selections.

▶ It alerts you to sugar content if you need or want to reduce your reliance on sweets.

▶ It is full of surprises. Sandwiches, spaghetti, and even some sugar can still make up part of your mealtimes.

▶ It works best when used in conjunction with informed label reading and portion-size awareness.

▶ It provides a safe approach to weight loss and risk reduction for many serious health problems.

▶ It is an at-home reference as well as a handy, portable guide that will help you make wise food choices every day.

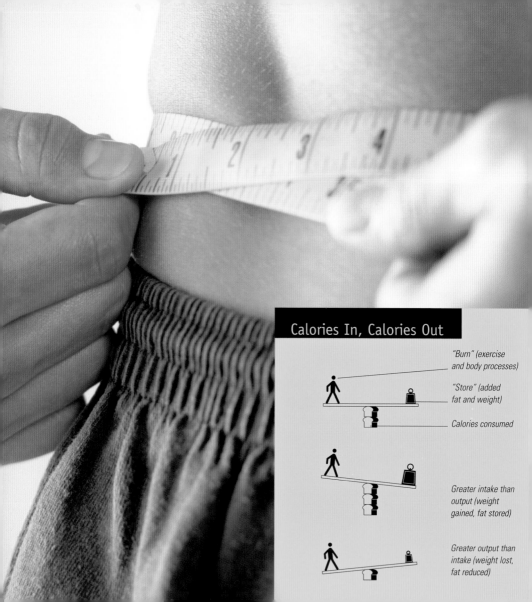

Calories In, Calories Out

"Burn" (exercise and body processes)

"Store" (added fat and weight)

Calories consumed

Greater intake than output (weight gained, fat stored)

Greater output than intake (weight lost, fat reduced)

4 The Big Picture

Clearly many people need to lose weight, but how can they do it successfully? Some look for the fastest way, others the easiest, still others want a way they know they'll be able to live with over the long haul. Researchers are currently trying to identify what is the most effective and long-lasting approach to weight loss that also reduces the risk of health problems associated with being overweight—without causing health problems of its own.

Weight-Loss Basics

The G.I. is a vital piece of the puzzle, but it is not the whole story. It's time to look at other factors that contribute to weight loss (and gain), as well as how the G.I. fits into the bigger picture—how it can help you lose weight, no matter what diet you try.

For years, conventional wisdom has stated that the way to lose weight is simply to take in fewer calories than you burn. Conversely, weight gain results from caloric intake that exceeds energy demands. This makes sense—except that it is evident that factors other than eating too much contribute to being overweight in far too many people. Moreover, calorie reduction does not always result in weight loss, as any dieter who has hit a "plateau" can attest.

Attempts have been made to explain the plateau phenomenon in terms of the "set point," the ill effects of "yo-yo" weight loss, and various other quasi-scientific theories. However, the bottom line is that people are not losing weight and keeping it off.

Burn it or store it: If you take in more calories than you need, your body will store it and you will gain weight. Eat less or exercise more, and you'll lose weight.

Calorie Theory vs. Metabolism Theory

Calories *do* count, but that's only part of the big picture. The body sometimes reacts to reduced calorie intake in ways that seem counterproductive. It stems from a primitive response to what feels like famine conditions. When calorie intake doesn't meet energy needs, fat is withdrawn from storage and converted to burnable form. The result is weight loss. After a while, the body gets the message that the calorie deficit may go on indefinitely and end in starvation. As a survival tactic, the metabolism slows down so it requires less fuel to keep the machine running. In short, it *adjusts* to make do with fewer calories. That's your "plateau," or "set point." It may have saved our Paleolithic ancestors when food was scarce, but it's no friend to today's dieter.

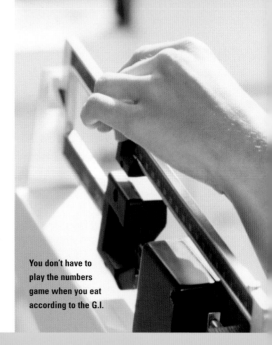

You don't have to play the numbers game when you eat according to the G.I.

It Explains a Lot

Seeing weight loss and weight gain as a combination of the calorie and metabolism theories makes sense of many mysteries, such as:

▶ Why some foods promote fat storage when different foods with the same caloric value do not.

▶ Why some foods produce hunger and cravings while others are more satisfying, even if their caloric values are similar.

▶ Why weight loss is more difficult for the very people who need it most: those who are obese or have diabetes or prediabetic conditions.

▶ Why exercise results in weight loss that exceeds the number of calories burned by the activity.

▶ Why it is relatively quick and easy to lose the first ten pounds and then discouragingly difficult, if not impossible, to lose more than that.

The *gi* Handbook

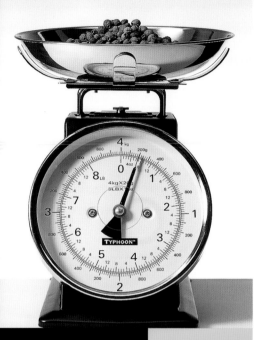

How Much Fuel?

Every gram of	Provides this many calories
Carbohydrate	4
Protein	4
Fat	9

How Much is a Gram?

Not much. It takes about 28 of them to add up to an ounce.

The Numbers

So is it just a matter of calories? No. The effect on insulin secretion and subsequent fat storage, the rate of digestion, and the many facets of metabolism all contribute to what happens to calories (in the form of food) once you swallow. The glycemic index, glycemic load, serving size, and level of physical activity are variables that must also be taken into account *in addition to* the calorie content of the food you eat.

Dieting is usually a minefield of numbers: calories, points, grams, B.M.I., and of course, pounds. It's good to know what some of these are and where they fit, but not to become obsessed with them.

Stop Playing the Numbers Game

Although the G.I. uses numbers to rank foods in comparison to glucose, there are too many variables to make sense of these in the real world outside the laboratory. Differences in a given person's health and metabolism are just the beginning of it. Processing and cooking methods, the effects of fat and protein eaten in combination with carbohydrates, even growing conditions and time of harvest change the G.I. value of a food to some degree. Moreover, obsessive number crunching leads to frustration, which leads to quitting.

The same goes for glycemic load. That is why we talk about G.I. in terms of ranges: *high*, *medium*, and *low*, as well as *none*—no G.I. at all. If you stay within the low to medium range and pay attention to your serving size, you can happily throw away your calculator.

If Weight Loss Were Easy, We'd All Be Slim

Even in the face of an avalanche of diet books and diet plans, too many of us are tipping the scales into obesity. Clearly, there is something wrong with this picture. Just as there is more to weight gain than just calories, there is more to weight loss than just dieting. A lot of what goes into our mouths has to do with what goes on in our heads. That comes as no surprise to anyone who has battled late-night cravings or hungered for comfort food when things weren't going smoothly. The question is: What can you do about it?

Emotional Eating

Left to their own devices, very young children will eat only as much as they need. As we get older, something happens to change our response to food. We eat to comfort or distract ourselves, to please others, to celebrate, to ease social encounters—and for many other reasons that have nothing to do with hunger or nutritional needs. We may begin eating because we are hungry, but then forget to stop. We eat too fast to notice we are sated. Often we take a second helping because we like the taste, we don't want to waste food, or just because that is our habit. We might have

Mindful Eating

One of the best strategies for conquering emotional eating is to heighten your awareness when you eat. If you can adopt even a few of the following habits, you may be on your way back to that childlike state of eating only as much as you need.

▸ Don't watch TV, read, or talk on the phone while eating.

▸ Fill your plate in the kitchen, then carry it into another room.

▸ Eat slowly, savoring each bite.

▸ If you want a snack, place a portion in a small bowl or plate and don't go back for a refill.

▸ Keep tempting but forbidden foods out of your house. If you cannot, put them out of reach and out of sight.

▸ Never eat standing up, especially not in front of an open refrigerator.

▸ When you cook, don't nibble or taste more than necessary.

▸ If you are hungry between meals, drink a glass of water or a cup of tea, then ask yourself if you really need to eat.

▸ Include low-G.I. carbohydrates in every meal and snack. They will satisfy your hunger and help you feel fuller for longer.

The *gi* Handbook

had a drink and our good intentions have flown along with our inhibitions. We might eat because we're depressed or anxious. We might use food as a reward or, conversely, overeat as a form of self-punishment.

Individual eating behavior is too complex to explore deeply here, but you can explore it on your own. Keep a food journal (*see pages 112–113*) and note how you feel before and after you have something to eat, as well as how long it's been since you last ate. You may notice patterns, triggers, and circumstances that cause you to eat more, or more often, than you should.

Set Some Goals

Our society blames and shames people who are overweight, and many blame themselves. Neither is helpful. It is time to get real: If you are overweight, you need to deal with it—for the sake of your health above everything else. So set some goals, and when you achieve them, raise the bar. Don't go for goals that have failure built into them. Be realistic about what and when you will eat, how much exercise you will get each day, and how much weight you intend to lose over a reasonable amount of time. You will have lapses. When that happens, try to understand what wasn't working, and get right back into the groove. Don't use a slip as an excuse for giving up.

Ask yourself: Are you really hungry or are you just thirsting for something sweet?

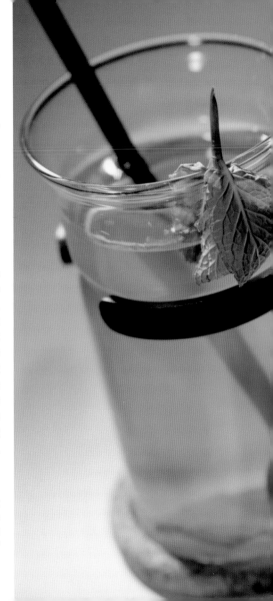

Nutrition 101

Once upon a time, there were four major food groups—dairy, meat, fruits and vegetables, and bread and cereal—and we were taught in school that eating some from each group would add up to a balanced diet. A simple rule for simpler times. Nutrition guidelines have gotten more complicated, but it's likely that most people do not understand today's guidelines and, therefore, do not follow them. Sadly, the old joke that the four food groups consist of "canned, frozen, takeout, and junk" paints a more realistic picture of what many people now eat. At the other end of the spectrum are diets that restrict entire classes of foods or tip the balance too far in one direction. We need all three macronutrients to fuel our bodies, and we need the micronutrients—vitamins and minerals—that are found in their most usable form in food, not in pills. We also need water, without which we would die long before we'd succumb to starvation. You already know how much carbohydrate, protein, and fat you need, and why. Now it's time to look at the other components of a healthy diet.

Carbohydrates of all kinds occupy the widest part of the food pyramid.

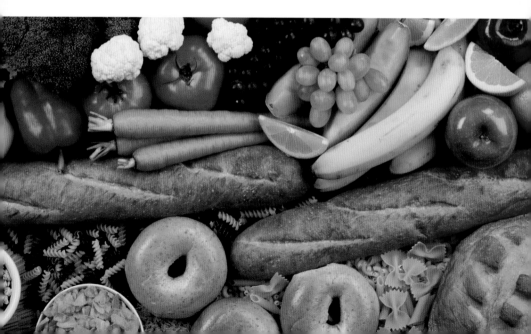

Is the Food Pyramid Ancient History?

Fifteen years after the food guide pyramid was unveiled, the venerable structure is undergoing renovations. Intended as an easy-to-understand graphic representation of the officially sanctioned balanced diet, the pyramid has fallen on hard times. The fact is, the eating public has never really understood it. More seriously, as a guide to making food choices, it has collapsed under the weight of the low-carb trend. Unfortunately for the builders of the pyramid, carbs are its foundation. True, sugar is banished from the wide base of the pyramid, scattered as small flakes at the tip and elsewhere throughout, but between the broad base of breads, cereals, rice, and pasta and the next level of fruits and vegetables, carbohydrates occupy the most prominent part of the structure.

Not surprisingly, carbs are at the center of the debate raging within the U.S. government's Dietary Guidelines Advisory Committee, and sugar is definitely the eye of the hurricane. On one side are countless studies that attribute being overweight or obese to increased consumption of sugar, especially in soft drinks. On the other side is the sugar industry, a powerful lobby that has gotten the anti-sugar message softened over the years. Other lobbying groups are weighing in with their own special interests. Many public health experts expect the new dietary recommendations will be stronger on politics than on nutrition.

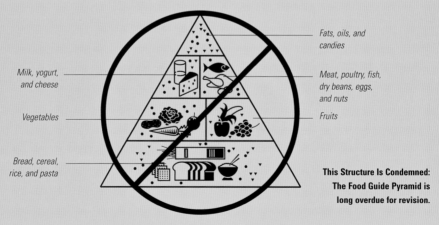

Fats, oils, and candies

Milk, yogurt, and cheese

Meat, poultry, fish, dry beans, eggs, and nuts

Vegetables

Fruits

Bread, cereal, rice, and pasta

**This Structure Is Condemned:
The Food Guide Pyramid is
long overdue for revision.**

The Small Picture

Vitamins and minerals are called micronutrients because we need only tiny amounts of them. But they pack a lot of power and are essential to every aspect of metabolism and body maintenance. Too little or, in some cases, too much can cause disease, disability, and deformity. Relying on supplements to be sure you get what you need may sound like a reasonable strategy, but the fact is food contains the necessary micronutrients in the form your body can use most efficiently. Fresh fruits and vegetables, dried beans, and unprocessed grains are among the best sources of many vitamins and minerals. They also happen to be low- and medium-G.I. foods.

Exceptions to the Rule

At various times of their lives, women have micronutrient needs that may not be entirely satisfied by food. During childbearing years they need extra folic acid to guard against serious birth defects that occur in the earliest stage of pregnancy. Many cereal and grain products are now fortified with folic acid. Women of all ages need calcium to keep their bones strong. After menopause, however, their calcium needs increase. Additional calcium is recommended for women on weight-loss diets. The body needs vitamin D to convert calcium to usable form, which is why this vitamin-mineral combination is often found in a single pill.

Minerals Matter

And there are many of them, far too many to list. Seven are considered "major" minerals, those we need 100 mg or more of each day. Thirteen others are considered "trace" minerals because we require exceedingly small amounts of them. Except for calcium, which women may need to supplement, you can get as much as you need by eating low- and medium-G.I. foods.

Major	Trace
▶ Calcium	▶ Chromium
▶ Chlorine	▶ Cobalt
▶ Magnesium	▶ Copper
▶ Phosphorus	▶ Fluorine
▶ Potassium	▶ Iodine
▶ Sodium	▶ Iron
▶ Sulfur	▶ Manganese
	▶ Molybdenum
	▶ Selenium
	▶ Silicon
	▶ Tin
	▶ Vanadium
	▶ Zinc

Vitamins Are Vital

Here's a brief rundown of the vitamins you need, together with their medium-, low-, and no-G.I. sources.

▶ A (beta-carotene, retinol, retinoic acid)	carrots, sweet potatoes, red peppers, green leafy vegetables, orange and red fruits, liver, eggs, and some fortified foods (read the label)
▶ B_1 (thiamin)	dried beans, whole grains, nuts, seeds, meat (especially pork)
▶ B_2 (riboflavin)	milk and dairy products (especially eggs and yogurt), liver, enriched breads and cereals (read the label)
▶ B_3 (niacin)	green leafy vegetables, dried beans, whole grains, nuts, seeds, fish, eggs, poultry, meat (especially liver)
▶ B_6 (pyridoxine)	green leafy vegetables, whole grains, dried beans, meat, fish
▶ B_{12} (cobalamin)	dairy (eggs, milk, cheese), meat, fish and shellfish, poultry
▶ Biotin (vitamin H)	whole grains, nuts, soybeans and soy products, mushrooms, liver
▶ C (ascorbic acid)	citrus fruit, berries, kiwi, melon, mango, papaya, tomato, peppers, and leafy green vegetables
▶ D	liver, eggs, fortified dairy products—also occurs naturally in sunlight
▶ E	nuts, whole grains, wheat germ, green leafy vegetables, vegetable and seed oils
▶ Folate (folic acid, folacin)	asparagus, spinach, and other leafy greens; dried beans, seeds; enriched or fortified breads, cereals, pasta, and orange juice (read the label)
▶ K	broccoli, brussels sprouts, cabbage, kale and other leafy greens; green tea; seaweed—also made in the body
▶ Pantothenic acid	eggs, kidneys, liver

Raise Your Carb Consciousness

The trouble with no-carb/low-carb diets is that they throw out the baby with the bath water, so to speak. It is both unwise and unhealthy to indiscriminately lump carbohydrates together and then ban them or reduce them to levels that are insufficient for the body's needs.

Instead, you can use the G.I. to tell you which carbohydrates to reduce or avoid, and which should be part of a well-balanced diet.

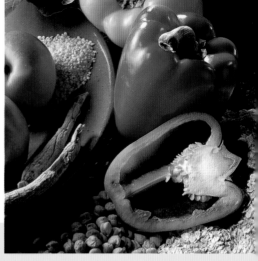

Know Your Carbs

Rather than putting all carbs on your blacklist, think of them in terms of ones you can eat *often*, *sometimes*, and *rarely*. Check the food lists in Chapter 6 for specifics.

Make whole grains, beans, and nonstarchy vegetables your everyday carbs.

Often	Sometimes	Rarely
Beans and other legumes	Canned fruit	Baked goods, such as cakes and cookies
Herbs	Dried fruit, such as apricots, prunes, and raisins	Candy and other sweets
Most fresh fruit	Fresh fruit such as bananas and cantaloupe	Refined grain products, such as breakfast cereals and bread
Nonstarchy vegetables	Ice cream	
Nuts and nut butters	Sugar and other sweeteners	Root and starchy vegetables, such as potatoes and rutabagas
Pasta	Whole-grain breads	
Salad and other greens	Whole-grain breakfast cereals	Snack foods, such as crackers and chips
Whole grains such as barley, buckwheat, and bulgur	Whole grains such as rice and cornmeal	Sweetened soft drinks

Fabulous Fiber

Cutting carbs often means losing the benefits of fiber. That makes no sense any way you look at it. Fiber is a calorie-free, fat-free wonder. You won't find it in oils or protein, but you will find it in abundance in foods that are also gold mines of vitamins and minerals. Soluble fiber slows digestion, which effectively lowers the G.I. of foods that contain it at the same time as helping you feel sated. It also helps lower LDL (*see pages 42–43*). Insoluble fiber absorbs water, adding bulk as it passes through your system. Not only does that keep you feeling fuller longer, it also promotes bowel regularity and prevents constipation, which appears to protect against diseases and disorders of the digestive system (ranging from diverticulosis and irritable bowel syndrome to cancer). Both types of fiber slow the absorption of glucose, which keeps your blood sugar levels low and steady. Many foods contain more than one kind of fiber and, best of all, most sources of fiber are also low G.I.

What You Miss When You Cut Carbs

▶ Essential brain food
▶ Natural sources of many vitamins and minerals
▶ Fiber
▶ Water—fat has none, protein has hardly any
▶ Satisfying bulk
▶ The most accessible form of energy to run your body

There are many good reasons why you should make sure 55 percent of your daily calorie intake is made up of carbohydrates. Indeed, they are irreplaceable.

Fiber-Rich Foods

Soluble
Fruit, including:
  Apples
  Grapefruit
  Grapes
  Oranges
  Peaches
  Pears
  Plums
  Prunes
Grains, including:
  Barley
  Oats
  Rye
Legumes, including:
  Beans of all kinds
  Lentils
Nuts and Seeds

Insoluble
Fruit, including:
  Apples
  Pears
Grains, including:
  Bran
  Germ
  Whole grains
Vegetables, including:
  Broccoli
  Cabbage
  Carrots
  Green beans
  Lettuce and other
  salad greens
  Peas
  Tomatoes

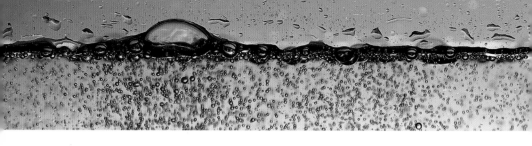

What About Water?

Believe it or not, more than half of you is made of water. That includes not only your blood, sweat, and tears, but also the fluid contents of every cell in your body. You can't live without it, but are you getting enough of it?

We get most of our water simply by drinking it, straight or in beverages. The rest comes in food. The standard advice is to drink 8 cups a day, but for most of us, that isn't enough. Adult males need about 13 cups and females about 9. The more active you are, the more water you need.

If you get most of your water by drinking sweetened beverages, you are taking on calories and glycemic load without gaining much nutritionally. Juices and soft drinks are essentially sugar water. Moreover, they are not as filling as solid food with the same G.I. and the same number of calories.

It's a better idea to fulfill more of your fluid requirements from plain drinking water, which provides important minerals, but no calories and no sugar, and to supplement it with solid fruits and vegetables, which have more staying power, not to mention quite a bit of water, vitamins, minerals, and lots of fiber.

Are you getting enough water? Most of us need more than we think...and drink.

The Big Fat Question

Somewhere amid the low-carb babble the idea has arisen that fat doesn't matter. Fat *does* matter—a lot. Fat may not raise blood sugar levels, but that does not mean it has no effect on weight and health.

No matter what kind of fat you eat, it has more than twice as many calories as an equal amount of carbohydrate or protein. That's twice as many calories for you to use or store.

Unsaturated fats—the kind found in vegetable, nut, and seed oils—carry health benefits along with their calorie load, so it makes sense to get most of your daily fat allowance from them. Saturated fat—the kind found in meat and dairy products—contributes to unhealthy levels of cholesterol, so it's best to keep your consumption of saturated fat to a minimum. Trans fat—found in everything from bottled salad dressings and bakery goods to snack foods and fried fast foods—deserve their bad reputation. The best way to avoid them is to read food labels and just say "no."

Exercise Is Not Optional

If you think exercise and dieting occupy two separate areas of your life, think again. If you want to lose weight, they must go hand in hand. The good news is that physical exercise is the answer to both the frustrating plateau periods during a diet and the "rebound effect" that too many of us experience once we have lost some weight and stop watching what we eat.

Regular exercise is the best way to counteract the metabolic slowdown that comes when your body is faced with the "famine" conditions of a diet. A half hour of even moderate exercise speeds up your metabolism for more than an hour afterward, so you keep burning calories even after you've stopped sweating. We know that follow-up studies of people who have lost weight through various diets have been discouraging, but the people who successfully maintained their weight loss were those who continued to exercise.

Experts recommend 30 minutes of moderate exercise at least five times a week.

Benefits All Around

Being physically active is the best thing you can do for yourself if you want to have a long and healthy life. The ideal combination improves strength, endurance, flexibility, and balance.

▶ Any kind of physical activity increases your body's energy demands, which burns calories.

▶ Physical activity speeds up your metabolism during and after exercise.

▶ Exercise that gets your heart pumping and makes you breathe faster conditions your heart, lungs, and circulatory system.

▶ Exercise that involves weights or resistance builds and maintains muscle mass.

▶ Weight-bearing exercise (including walking) builds and maintains bone mass, delaying or even preventing the development of osteoporosis.

▶ All physical activity increases levels of brain chemicals to give you an emotional boost. It is a highly effective natural antidepressant.

▶ Exercise reduces stress, which in turn reduces the risk of both physical and emotional ills.

▶ Engaging in physical activity with friends and family enriches your social life and is just plain fun.

No Matter What Diet

The G.I. is not a diet, but it is the scientific basis of some of today's most popular weight-loss ideas. In order to grab headlines and book sales, a diet has to have a special "twist." Now that you understand so much about metabolism, you will be able to look beyond the hype and recognize that the general focus on carbohydrates is really about how quickly they are broken down into glucose and the speed and degree to which they cause insulin levels to rise. That will allow you to choose a diet that makes sense and will work for you—your tastes, your temperament, and your lifestyle.

Is It Safe?

To safeguard your health, take these steps before you embark on any diet:

▶ Avoid diets that encourage an overload of fat, especially of saturated and trans fats.

▶ Be aware that extremely high protein diets may stress your kidneys.

▶ Make sure the diet does not leave you deficient in vitamins and minerals.

▶ Remember that you need *a minimum* of 150 grams of carbohydrates daily.

▶ If in doubt, ask your doctor, especially if you are being treated for any sort of health problem.

Taking Sides

Arguments rage about which "low-carb" diet is better, easier to live with, more effective, and more enduring. These disputes rely on what researchers call anecdotal evidence rather than on scientific proof. Proof requires well-designed and controlled clinical studies that compare the diets head to head. No one has done that, and no one is likely to anytime soon. The closest anyone has come was a short study comparing the Atkins diet (low-carbohydrate, high-protein, high-fat) with a low-calorie, high-carb, low-fat diet. The conclusion? Dieters did equally poorly when it came to sticking with the diet and maintaining weight loss. Neither diet used the G.I. in selecting the carb component. In the absence of conclusive studies, don't take sides. Instead, raise your "carb consciousness" and use the G.I. to ensure you get enough of the right kind of carbohydrates, no matter which diet you choose.

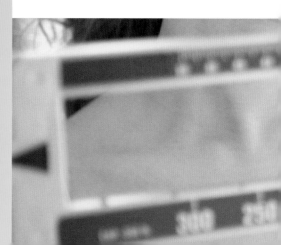

The Diets A–Z

There are dozens of carb-conscious diets in vogue today and many more are sure to be introduced in the future. Some of these are sounder than others; all can be made easier and safer to follow by using the G.I. to aid your food choices and to broaden the selection of permissible carbohydrate foods. Here's a brief rundown on nine diets that are currently the most popular.

The Atkins Diet

This is the 800-pound gorilla of low-carb diets. It's been around for more than 30 years, though Dr. Robert Atkins eventually loosened his original near-total ban on carbs to permit a gradual reintroduction of this important macronutrient as adherents near their weight-loss goals. This four-stage diet, which purports to be a lifetime eating plan, recognizes the connection between carbohydrates and insulin in fat metabolism, but it is potentially high in saturated fat and deficient in vitamins and minerals, unless non-carb foods are chosen with great care. Modifying the Atkins Diet with a good knowledge of the glycemic index could make it safer, but no less effective in the long run.

The Carbohydrate Addict's Diet

Rachael and Richard Heller's approach to diet combines the sound science of the carb-insulin-fat relationship with a questionable theory that addictive cravings are caused by an interaction between insulin and serotonin, which is an important brain chemical. Following this highly prescriptive diet is quite complicated. It can be simplified by using the G.I. to choose permitted carbohydrates for both the "complementary" (low-G.I.) meals and the "reward" meal, a once-daily free choice event that allows high-G.I. foods.

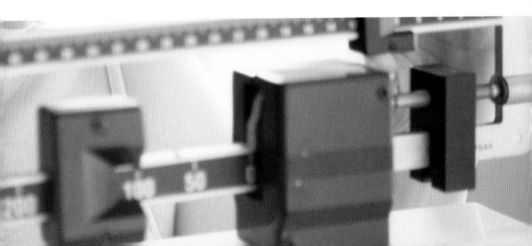

Cave Man Diets

Not a single diet, this group includes "Neanderthin" and the "Paleo Diet." The premise is that we'd all be better off eating like our hunter-gatherer ancestors. Admirably, these diets exclude refined and processed foods; inexplicably, they also forbid whole grains, legumes, and dairy of all kinds. There is a potential for vitamin and mineral deficiency as well as inadequate intake of carbohydrates, especially fiber. Adding high-fiber and low- to medium-G.I. foods might spoil the prehistoric gimmick, but it will make for a healthier eating plan.

The Fat Flush Plan

Whether or not you believe the liver will metabolize fat more effectively if it is "flushed" of toxins, the basis of this particular diet is a healthy balance of low-fat protein, unsaturated fat, and low-G.I. carbohydrates, which add up to a calorie-controlled regimen—and it is quite regimented. Carbohydrate

intake is gradually increased over three phases. You may find this diet easier to stick with if you use the G.I. to supplement the list of "friendly carbs."

The Glucose Revolution

This is the original "orthodox" G.I.-based diet. After reading *The G.I. Handbook*, you will find no surprises in this diet or any of the series of books that are designed to guide you through it. It is important to note that weight loss depends on restricting caloric intake *as well as* eating food that is consistently low on the G.I.

Protein Power

Anyone who understands the nutritional importance of carbohydrates will be alarmed by the extreme restriction this diet imposes. The first of three phases allows no more than 30 grams of carbohydrates per day, which increases to 55 in phase two, and then in 10-gram increments in phase three as long as your

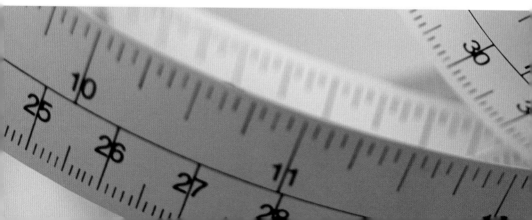

weight remains stable. That's a long time to be starved of needed carbs. Meanwhile, protein intake is far in excess of what is needed and invites high fat (especially saturated fat) intake as well. The plan involves "effective" carbs—subtracting fiber from the total carbohydrate content. This over-simplification of the G.I. robs dieters of the body fuel they need.

The South Beach Diet

There's a reason why this diet is so popular: It's a common sense, balanced approach to eating to lose weight and reduce health risks. After a quick weight-loss phase that severely restricts carbs, it allows them to take their proper place in a balanced eating plan. Dr. Arthur Agatston stresses the distinction between "good" and "bad" carbs. The basis for this is, of course, the G.I. That makes it an excellent tool to use in phases two and three—especially as the latter is meant to last for the rest of your life.

Sugar Busters!

As the name suggests, this diet demonizes sugar. It is otherwise based on the principles of the G.I., bolstered with portion control to add up to a reasonably balanced diet. The authors, all M.D.s, recognize the role of insulin in both health and disease. Because it is not a structured weight-loss regimen, it requires anyone who follows it to do a lot of planning. The G.I. should be central to that task.

The Zone

This popular diet stresses overall health more than weight loss and gives insulin its due. In fact, the "zone" refers to a low, smooth insulin curve. With its daily allotment of 40 percent carbohydrates and 30 percent each for fat and protein, it allows more carbs than most carb-conscious diets, but still not as many as we need. Using the G.I. makes it possible to increase carbohydrate intake without falling out of the "zone."

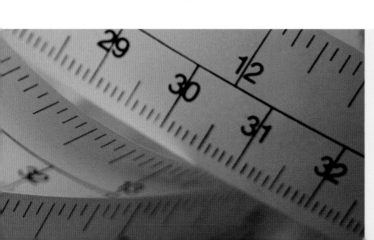

Some diets leave you carb-starved or fat-saturated. Use what you have learned to make wiser choices.

Lifetime Lifestyle

Rather than diets, what we really need is a whole new lifestyle. We should eat sensibly and get more exercise—starting today and for the rest of our lives. Diets are hard work. They are boring. They are discouraging. And they do not last. The G.I. is an approach to eating that works because it is practical, easy to follow, and is based on solid science. It provides a wide variety of choices so that you can eat food you like without feeling hungry or deprived. It provides you with the fuel your body needs so that you will have the energy to be more active. It is, in short, the kind of lifestyle change that will make a lifelong difference.

Long-term lifestyle changes are healthier for you than off-and-on dieting.

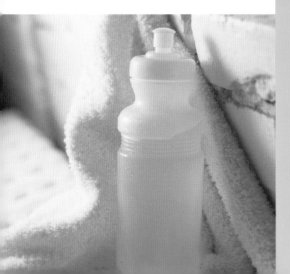

Feeling Better About Feeling Good

The prospect of losing weight and exercising more can be daunting. A lot of us feel defeated even before we begin. But here's some good news to motivate you to start, and to keep on going.

▶ No matter how much you weigh, a loss of as little as 5–10 percent can reduce your risk of diabetes and heart disease.

▶ If you start by trading one high-G.I. food for a medium- or low-G.I. choice each day, you can effortlessly reshape your eating habits over time.

▶ As little as 30 minutes of moderate exercise, such as walking three days a week, can put you on the road to better health.

▶ You don't have to get your daily exercise in a single session. Ten-minute bursts of activity are just as effective as one longer session.

▶ Every step you take in the direction of weighing less and being more active puts more distance between you and the risks that threaten your health and life.

Begin with modest goals. You will be surprised what a big difference a few small changes can make.

Summing Up: The Big Picture

- When it comes to weight loss, both calories and metabolism play a part.

- Taking in more calories than you use will always result in weight gain.

- Reducing caloric intake may not result in weight loss if your body adjusts by lowering its metabolic demand.

- Regular physical activity is the most effective way to raise metabolic demand so that you burn more than you store.

- Food is the best source of vitamins and minerals, and carbohydrates are the richest source of these essential micronutrients.

- The G.I. helps you to get the benefits of carbohydrates without the blood sugar ups and downs.

- Changing your behavior and attitudes toward food is vital if you want to lose weight and keep it off.

- Success depends on setting realistic goals and gradually raising the bar.

- Combining the G.I. with portion control, behavioral change, and exercise is the best way to ensure weight loss that lasts.

- It's easy to use the G.I. if you think in terms of foods you should eat: *often*, *sometimes*, and *rarely*.

- The G.I. can be used with any carb-conscious diet to ensure you get enough of the right kind of carbohydrates.

- The G.I. is the cornerstone of a lifetime eating plan.

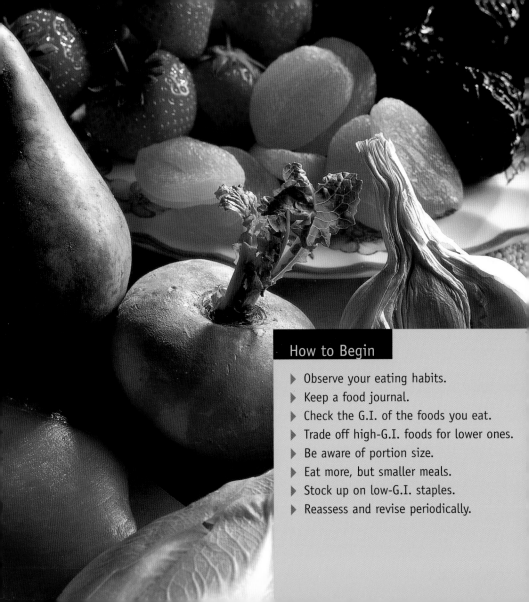

How to Begin

▶ Observe your eating habits.
▶ Keep a food journal.
▶ Check the G.I. of the foods you eat.
▶ Trade off high-G.I. foods for lower ones.
▶ Be aware of portion size.
▶ Eat more, but smaller meals.
▶ Stock up on low-G.I. staples.
▶ Reassess and revise periodically.

5 The G.I. Way to Healthy Living

The G.I. allows you to choose from a wide variety of foods that are among the healthiest around, the richest sources of vitamins and minerals, phytochemicals, and fiber. By keeping your blood sugar levels in check, a low-G.I. diet helps guard against many health risks, including being overweight and diabetes. The G.I. does not, however, give you *carte blanche* to eat as much as you like.

Strategic Thinking

A huge portion of low-G.I. food has the potential to raise your blood sugar as much as a tiny taste of a high-G.I. food. That's because glycemic load— G.I. multiplied by carb grams (*see page 75*)— determines how much glucose ends up in your blood. You can read all the food labels you like, but if you double the amount you eat and don't take into account the fact that you are also doubling the carbohydrates, not to mention the calories, sugar, and fat, you are fooling only yourself.

Whether you want to lose weight or lower your risk of diabetes and heart problems, you can take a giant step on the way to healthy living by using the G.I. to guide your food choices. Begin by monitoring your eating habits: when you feel hungry and when you are sated; whether you eat when you're hungry or bored; and above all, how much you eat. Next, make a list of what foods you eat and use the food lists in Chapter 6 to determine the G.I. range. Try to replace high-G.I. foods with medium- to low-G.I. ones. Aim for one substitution per day until high G.I. is the exception, not the rule.

It's easy to find low- and medium-G.I. replacements to break your high-G.I. habits.

They Call It "Portion Distortion"

According to the National Institutes of Health, America's weight is out of control because people have no idea how much they eat. Over the past two decades, food and drink portions have mushroomed. An individual container of soda used to be 8 ounces—now it's 12, and many fast-food restaurants pour out a super-size 20 or 44 ounces. Movie houses sell giant tubs of buttered popcorn along with huge soft drinks, and then offer free refills. Bagels once measured about 3 inches and 130 calories. Now they've ballooned to 6 inches or more, and typically weigh in at 350 calories. It takes a lot of cream cheese to cover all that territory. Muffins have undergone a similar transformation, growing bigger and sweeter over time. Even a quarter-pound hamburger was nearly twice the recommended serving, but now people are eating double burgers with an extra piece of bun between them. Today's portion of french fries is close to three times as large as it was 20 years ago, and who remembers that a serving of pasta is supposed to be 2 ounces out of the box, a cup on the plate? Between "salad" bars and all-you-can-eat buffets, people have gotten into the habit of filling their plates to overflowing and then going back for seconds. No wonder the NIH calls it portion distortion!

Portion Control Tools

Keep these items handy and use them until you get a feel for what a serving looks like:

▶ Kitchen scale

▶ Measuring cups

▶ Measuring spoons

When you're away from home, use your eyes:

▶ A 3-ounce serving of meat, fish, or poultry is the size of a deck of cards.

▶ A half cup of rice or ice cream would fill half a tennis ball; a cup of pasta would fill a whole one.

▶ A tablespoon of jam is no bigger than a gameboard checker.

▶ Your stomach is about the size of your fist—think about that each time you fill your plate.

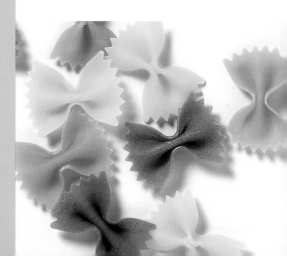

To complicate matters, the official government position on what constitutes a serving often differs from that of food manufacturers. For example, according to the USDA, a serving of ready-to-eat cereal is 1 ounce; most cereal labels show twice that amount. The label reads 8 ounces, whereas the USDA calls 6 ounces a serving of fruit or vegetable juice. More static from the Tower of Babel. If you're trying to match calorie and nutrient content with serving size, the food label is probably your best source of information.

Journalese

Most of us have no idea how much we eat on any given day. We may pay attention to what we eat at mealtimes, but all those in-betweens are easy to forget. Getting it all down on paper may help you focus and keep your eyes on the prize. Make copies of the blank journal on pages 112–113 or design your own. Try it for a month, or longer if it works for you.

Write down everything you eat, including those nibbles or whatever else you unconsciously put in your mouth in the course of a day. You may be amazed.

Weights and Measures

Success is a great motivator. So is a hard dose of reality. Aside from paying attention to what, when, and how much you eat, here are some other ways to keep yourself on track.

▶ Weigh yourself once a week, using the same scales. Write your weight on a calendar or in your journal.

▶ Figure out your B.M.I., using the chart on page 56. Repeat this once a month and write down any change. Your goal is to be between 18 and 24.

▶ Measure your waist (at the level of your navel) and write it down. Do it again in a month, and write down the new measurement. Your primary goal is less than 35 inches (women) and 40 inches (men). You set your secondary goal.

▶ Once a year, get a fasting blood lipid test (total cholesterol, HDL, and triglycerides). Blood pressure and blood sugar should also be tested annually. Ask for written records of the results. If you're outside the normal range, talk to your doctor about what steps to take.

Daily Food and Activity Journal

	Monday		Tuesday		Wednesday	
	Food	G.I.	Food	G.I.	Food	G.I.
Breakfast Time:						
Lunch Time:						
Dinner Time:						
Snack Time(s):						
Activity						

Goals: Diet   Physical activity

Behavior

Thursday		Friday		Saturday		Sunday	
Food	G.I.	Food	G.I.	Food	G.I.	Food	G.I.

Goals: Diet   Physical activity

Behavior

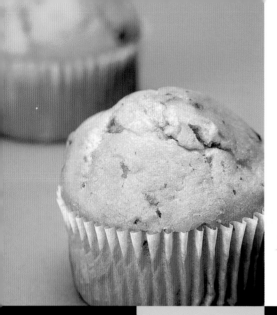

Eating the G.I. Way

You may have to say good-bye to french fries and sugar-laden cereal, but you can cook delicious meals and even entertain in style without straying into high-G.I. territory. All it takes is a little planning.

Consider the Possibilities

It's taken you a lifetime to develop your eating habits; don't try to change them overnight. The idea is to find delicious alternatives to the high-G.I. foods you have eaten in the past. If you make two or three substitutions a week, you'll be eating in a much healthier way before you know it. If you make one a day, all the better!

Instead of a donut, have an apple-oatmeal muffin.

Instead of...	Choose...
▶ Granola	▶ Oatmeal, with banana slices
▶ English muffin with strawberry jam	▶ Whole-grain toast with peaches and cottage cheese
▶ Fish and chips	▶ Shrimp scampi with fettuccine
▶ Hamburger and fries	▶ Chef's salad
▶ Potato salad and fried chicken	▶ Three-bean salad and grilled chicken kabobs
▶ Pie à la mode	▶ Strawberries dipped in chocolate
▶ A frozen daiquiri	▶ A Bloody Mary
▶ Potato chips and sour cream-onion dip	▶ Raw vegetables and yogurt-mint dip
▶ Cola	▶ Ice tea

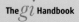

How Many Meals?

Traditionally—and theoretically—we eat three meals a day. In fact, many of us skip breakfast and make up for it with more snacks than we care to admit. It is time to discard the three meals model, but it has to be done rationally.

Studies have shown that multiple small meals are better than fewer large ones when it comes to modulating blood sugar levels and controlling hunger. Small meals also help you feel better because they don't leave you stuffed and sleepy, and they are a realistic way to deal with the fact that people do get hungry (or bored) more than three times a day. This new pattern has been called *grazing*, an unfortunate term because it implies constant consumption. The idea is to eat separate and distinct small meals according to a schedule that matches your personal hunger pattern. If you've spent time observing your eating habits, you should have a good idea what that pattern is. Give this new approach a try, and revise it if necessary. But remember, it's multiple small meals, so don't listen to the *multiple* and tune out the *small*. If your total daily consumption increases, so will your weight. So think about snack-size servings when you're the cook, and appetizers and half portions when you eat out.

A half portion of pasta makes a perfect mini-meal.

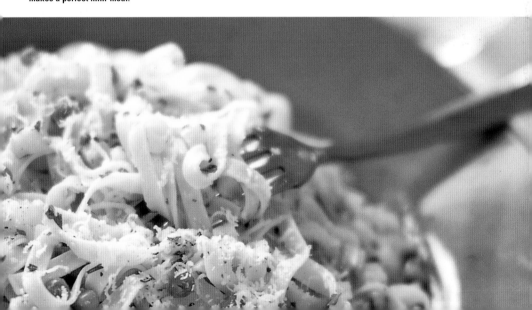

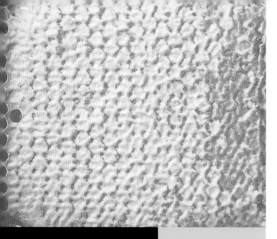

Sugar Surprises

When you look at the ingredient list on a label, be sure you know these sugar aliases.

- Barley malt
- Beet sugar
- Brown sugar
- Cane sugar
- Corn sweetener
- Corn syrup
- Date sugar
- Dextrose
- Fructose
- Fruit juice concentrate
- Glucose
- Honey
- Invert sugar
- Lactose
- Maltodextrins
- Maltose
- Maple sugar, syrup
- Molasses
- Raw sugar
- Sorghum
- Sucrose
- Turbinado sugar

Natural, refined, or in disguise—by any name, it's still sugar.

Shop Smart

The supermarket can be a minefield, but if you plan ahead, it can be a low-G.I. gold mine.

- Consult the food lists in Chapter 6 to plan your meals and snacks. If you need ideas, read on.

- Check what ingredients you already have on hand, then make a list of what you need.

- Take your list and *The G.I. Handbook* with you when you go shopping.

- If you are tempted by anything that is not on your list, check the G.I. before you buy.

- Read the labels, especially if you can't find the G.I. Watch out for saturated and trans fats, and sugar by any name.

In the Kitchen

Preparing meals the G.I. way can be as easy as opening a few containers or zapping something in the microwave. If you enjoy cooking, however, it provides a chance to be inventive. In many cases, you can adapt tried and true recipes by substituting lower G.I. ingredients. In others, a few additions will make a difference to the overall G.I. And in the case of two low-G.I. superstars—beans and barley (*see page 118*)—it's just a matter of knowing what to do with them.

▶ Broths and stocks: Buy them in cans or boxes, or make them yourself (*see below*). If you have to, use bouillon cubes, but be aware that they have more sugar and salt than you'd expect. Use broths and stocks as the base for soups or the liquid for cooking grains. Instead of flour-thickened gravies, make flavorful reductions and glazes. Simply boil down any broth or stock until it has a bold flavor—or even further until it becomes dark and syrupy.

▶ Herbs and spices: Flavorwise, these pack a lot of punch. The quantities you use are so small that they are all fat-, calorie-, and G.I.-free. So expand your collection and experiment with some new tastes.

▶ Soup bones, and so on: Beef, pork, and lamb bones make a richer stock if you oven-roast them first. Smoked ham bones and hocks are especially compatible with legumes. Fish heads and lobster shells make delicious seafood stock. Chicken and turkey carcasses cook down to a rich broth. Toss some carrots, onions, and celery into the pot, add water to cover, and simmer until it tastes good. Strain the solids and refrigerate the liquid for a few hours so

that you can lift off the layer of fat. For a ready supply of homemade bouillon cubes, boil down the strained stock until it is very concentrated, pour it into ice-cube trays, and when frozen, transfer to a freezer bag.

▶ Vinegar and citrus juice: It's a happy fact that acid lowers the G.I. of any food. So think beyond salad dressing. A squirt of these acidic liquids adds a bright flavor to cooked vegetables, pasta sauces, dips, grilled meats, and so on. Whether red or white, apple cider or malt, balsamic or herb-infused, all vinegar has zero G.I., calories, and fat. Instead of canned fruit cocktail in sugar syrup, make a lively fresh fruit salad with lime juice and fresh mint leaves. Add a tablespoon of tangerine juice to a meat glaze. Make a deliciously mysterious dip by thinning yogurt with a bit of orange juice and adding grated orange zest and a sprinkle of nutmeg.

▶ Wine: Add it to soups, stews, and sauces. The alcohol evaporates during cooking, leaving behind a deep, rich flavor.

Some Key Ingredients

Barley—Barley is low G.I. and high fiber, but often overlooked. Most of us think of it purely as a starchy soup ingredient. But barley is also a flavorful substitute for rice. As the food lists in Chapter 6 show, rice is all over the G.I. map. Arborio rice, used to make risotto, is high, and even brown rice is medium, while bland converted white rice and exotic japonica are low. Barley is an alternative to all of them and it makes a terrific risotto. Like arborio rice, it cooks into the thick oatmeal-like texture that is characteristic of risotto, but *without* a high G.I. rating. Just follow any risotto recipe, substituting barley measure for measure.

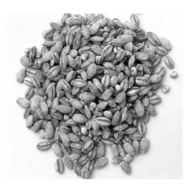

There are many other ways to cook with barley. For example, sauté some chopped onions in a bit of olive oil, then add the barley and stir until it's shiny with oil. Pour in twice as much water or broth as the barley and cook just as you would rice. Or spread the dry barley in a shallow pan and put it in the oven until golden brown, then cook it as though it were rice. The toasty flavor and chewy texture will have your family saying, "Let's have barley rather than rice."

Legumes—Legumes are universally low G.I. Though they tend to be bland, they are excellent vehicles for zesty herbs and spices. Many people shun dried beans and their ilk because of their gas-producing reputation. In fact, once your digestive system gets used to them, this is rarely a problem. It helps if you soak them overnight, discard the soaking water, and cook them in fresh water.

Channa dal, a dried legume resembling yellow split peas, is a staple in India but little known in the West. You may find it in some health and ethnic food stores. If you can't find it, ask for it. If enough people do, it may become a staple here, too. Its selling point is its rock-bottom G.I. But channa dal is not the only option. Split peas, lentils, and the vast range of beans are all as versatile as they are low G.I., high fiber, and nonfat sources of protein.

Cooked legumes can be made into spreads, dips, soups, and sauces. Toss them into salads instead of croutons, or try this alternative to popcorn and other high-G.I. nibbles: Spread cooked chickpeas or soybeans on a cookie sheet and bake them in a moderate oven until crisp. Add a little bit of salt if you like.

The water that beans have been cooked in makes a wonderful soup base. Toss in some herbs and aromatics. Sage, bay leaf, and rosemary are especially good for giving beans some depth of flavor; cooking any legume with onion, garlic, celery, and carrots yields a nice stock.

Yogurt "Cheese"—Plain, low-fat yogurt is remarkably versatile, especially if you thicken it by draining off most of the liquid whey. To do this, fit a round coffee filter into a sieve and place it over a bowl. Spoon yogurt into the filter and refrigerate for a few hours or overnight. Discard the whey or use it to make stock.

The yogurt will be the consistency of cream cheese, and smooth and tangy. Add a bit of garlic and some fresh chopped herbs to make a piquant spread, or thin it with fruit juice for a dip or dessert topping. Stir it into a vinaigrette for a creamy salad dressing. Top a bowl of tomato or puréed bean soup with a spoonful and scatter chopped chives or dill over the surface. Whisk it with reduced stock to make a creamy sauce or gravy for fish, meat, or chicken. In short, use this low-fat, low-G.I. alternative in any recipe that calls for sour or sweet cream, goat cheese, or crème fraîche.

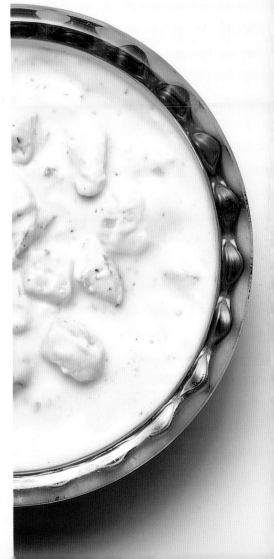

Drained low-fat yogurt "cheese" is a versatile stand-in when you want a creamy taste and texture without the fat.

What's on the Menu?

The possibilities are endless, but here are just a few ideas for meals throughout the day. For each, you will find a home-cooked menu and another option for when you are away from home—either brown-bagging it or ordering at a restaurant—plus a handful of other choices. Armed with your understanding of the G.I. principles and the food lists in Chapter 6, you will be able to mix and match, and come up with your own ideas, too.

Choose whole fruit over juice to get fiber along with your vitamins.

Breakfast

The biggest mistake dieters make is to skip breakfast. The way they see it, they're not that hungry and they can save time and calories. In fact, breakfast comes at the end of the longest interval between meals, whether you stop eating at dinner or have a midnight snack. Your blood sugar is low, your metabolism is slow, and your brain and body are in need of fuel. You need breakfast to start up the engine and get through the day. Carb-conscious dieters are especially prone to skipping this meal since so many breakfast foods are heavy on carbs and tend to be sweet. But there are many excellent low- and medium-G.I. choices, whether you "break your fast" at home or on your way to work.

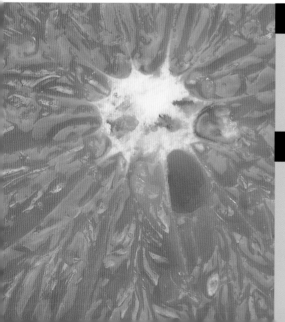

At Home

▶ Bran cereal with milk and raisins or sliced banana
▶ Half a grapefruit
▶ Coffee or tea

On the Go

▶ Breakfast egg salad sandwich made with a hard-boiled egg, one slice of crisp bacon crumbled, and a teaspoon of mayonnaise on whole-grain rye bread
▶ Orange sections
▶ Hot or iced latte

Other Options

▶ Whole-grain French toast topped with applesauce (made without sugar) and a dusting of cinnamon

▶ Yogurt smoothie, made from 1 cup of plain yogurt and ¼ cup of apple juice, blended with one or more of the following: pitted prunes, banana, strawberries, vanilla extract, malted milk powder, espresso coffee

▶ Home-baked bran-raisin muffin

▶ Cream of Wheat with raisins and sweetened soy milk

▶ Mixed fruit with flavored and sweetened yogurt topped with 2 tablespoons of All-Bran cereal

▶ Cottage cheese with either orange or grapefruit sections

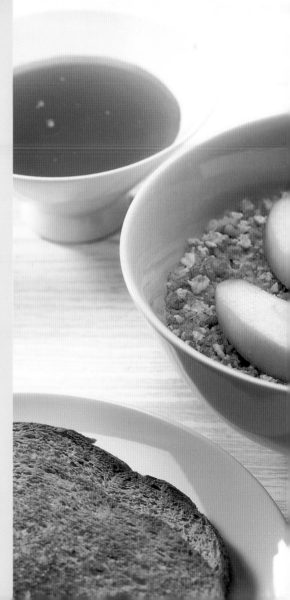

Oatmeal or other whole-grain cereal with fresh fruit is a better breakfast choice than supermarket "whole wheat" toast.

Lunch

Whether at home or away, lunch usually means a sandwich. But what if bread is off-limits? Soups and hearty salads with beans, hard-boiled eggs, water-packed tuna, and chicken cubes are excellent alternatives. But you don't have to give up on sandwiches. The key is dense, whole-grain bread. Look for the type with thin slices with visible grains. They are chewy and more flavorful than spongy "whole-grain" breads. If you opt for a softer bread, make an open-faced sandwich, using one slice instead of two.

At Home

- Chicken salad with ginger, scallions, celery, and sunflower seeds, bound with tahini and yogurt
- A slice of dense multi-grain bread
- Spiced tea with sweetened soy milk
- A fresh pear

On the Go

- Yogurt cheese on dense pumpernickel
- Cherry tomatoes and carrot sticks
- A glass of ice tea with mint
- A tangerine or clementine
- Two low- to medium-G.I. cookies

Other Options

- Soup: gazpacho, mushroom barley, tomato, lentil, or black bean
- Sandwich fillers: hummus, baba ghanoush (eggplant spread), peanut butter, canned fish (tuna, salmon, sardines), chicken or turkey breast, roasted peppers, alfalfa sprouts, olive spread, sun-dried tomato and pesto spread
- Salads: tabouli with tomatoes and cucumber, chef's salad with creamy yogurt vinaigrette, salade niçoise (lettuce, tuna, capers, cooked string beans, tomatoes); three-bean salad with minced scallions and mustardy vinaigrette, Greek salad with feta cheese, olives, and stuffed grape leaves

Start with salad, but don't stop there. There's a wealth of low-G.I. food on the menu.

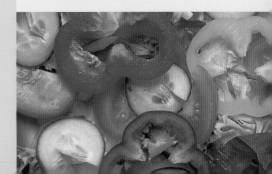

Dinner

The evening meal can be plain or fancy, a family gathering or a romantic dinner for two. Traditionally it is the biggest meal of the day, though there is no real reason why it should be. Too often the result is a profound sleepiness that drives us to the couch, remote control in one hand and a container of Cherry Garcia in the other. If you eat a multi-course dinner, consider following up with a brisk walk or other moderate exercise. You will be amazed how it banishes fatigue.

At Home

- Pasta with white clam sauce (clams and broth, white wine, olive oil, garlic, red pepper flakes, chopped parsley)
- Arugula, chickpeas, and roasted red peppers with balsamic vinaigrette
- A glass of wine or water
- Fresh fruit and one piece of almond biscotti

Dining Out

- Cup of soup du jour or house salad
- Grilled fish in lemon butter sauce with boiled new potatoes and string beans
- A glass of wine
- Chocolate mousse

Other Options

- Shrimp cocktail with ketchup-horseradish sauce and a squeeze of lemon juice
- Raw oysters with mignonette sauce
- Mixed green salad
- Caprese salad (tomato, mozzarella, and basil)
- Lentil, watercress, and Vidalia onion salad
- Jicama slaw with orange sections and orange juice-cumin dressing
- Barley seafood risotto (made with shellfish broth, minced onions or shallots, lemon juice and zest, and topped with shrimp, scallops, or other shellfish)
- Wild and white rice pilaf with wild mushrooms and braised veal with gremolata (orange and lemon zest chopped finely with parsley and garlic)
- Roast pork loin, baked apple slices dusted with nutmeg, and white turnips mashed with roasted garlic
- Spinach tortellini with ricotta and herbs
- Tofu and vegetable stir fry with sesame seeds on a bed of cellophane noodles
- Half a pear poached in port wine, half a scoop of vanilla ice cream, and a drizzle of poaching liquid reduced to syrup
- Pound cake

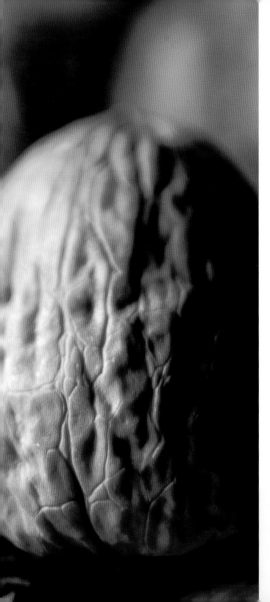

Snacks

A snack can be your best friend or your worst enemy. If you are noshing mindlessly because your relationship with food is out of control, it is time for a serious assessment of your weight, your health, and the emotional background to your overeating. If you gobble something down because you are famished, chances are you skipped breakfast or recently had a high-G.I. meal and are hungry because of a blood sugar/insulin rebound.

In both these cases, you may grab whatever is nearest at hand, and the likelihood is that it will be high G.I. and laden with sugar or fat, as most snack foods are. If, however, you have decided to eat multiple small meals each day and it is time for your mid-morning, mid-afternoon, or mid-evening snack, you will be reasonably hungry and ready to readjust your blood sugar level. Depending on the time of day, what else you have planned to eat that day, where you are, and your own preferences, the snack you choose may be sweet, salty, "hot," or bland.

The range of G.I.-safe choices is nearly endless. Start here and then check the food lists in Chapter 6 for more low- and medium-G.I. ideas on what to munch when you have the munchies.

A tough nut to crack? It's better than eating mixed nuts by the handful.

Snacking the G.I. Way

- A cup of soup
- Chai (hot or chilled) with a low-G.I. muffin
- Cherry tomatoes
- Chocolate bar
- Chocolate-covered peanuts: Count out 20 and put the rest away
- Chocolate malted soy milk smoothie
- Creamy salsa-yogurt dip with raw vegetables and homemade tortilla chips (cut a low-G.I. tortilla in eighths, then crisp the pieces in a toaster oven)
- Fruit-flavored yogurt, from the container, either blended as a smoothie or whipped and frozen
- Fresh fruit: Choose an apple, grapes, orange, pear, or plum
- Latte: hot, iced, or frozen; with a dusting of cinnamon, nutmeg, or chocolate powder
- Low- to medium-G.I. cookies with a piece of fruit or glass of milk
- Low-G.I. sports bar
- Nuts: You can keep fat and calories under control if you count out a reasonable number of nuts *in their shells* so you have to work at getting to them.
- Olives
- Open-faced sandwich on whole-grain bread with cheese and alfalfa sprouts
- Peanut butter on a celery stalk
- Raw vegetables and dip (hummus, baba ghanoush, guacamole, or a mustardy vinaigrette)
- Snack tortilla filled with shredded lettuce, black beans, guacamole, and salsa
- Strawberries dipped in melted bittersweet chocolate
- Stuffed grape leaves
- Trail mix made with soy or garbanzo "nuts," sunflower or pumpkin seeds, raisins, chopped dried apricots or apples
- Yogurt cheese on whole-wheat toast: Make it sweet or spicy.

Cooking for Kids

If you have children, you know how important it is to shepherd them through their childhood safely and in good health. Physical activity and good eating habits are the best safeguards against becoming overweight and the serious health problems that are associated with that.

As long as they are under your roof, you will be able to influence your children's diet—at least to some degree (*see also page 129*). You may have to combat peer pressure, aggressive advertising, and ever-present junk food, but if you can manage to make low- and medium-G.I. choices palatable and interesting, you'll improve the chances of winning the battle.

One of the best ways to get kids to buy into a healthy diet is to involve them in the choices and preparation of the food they eat. You can start doing this when children are quite young, taking them to the supermarket and talking about what you are buying and why you are doing so. As they get older, plan snacks and meals that kids can assemble or help you prepare. Even picky eaters can be tempted by G.I.-safe foods.

Child-Friendly Foods

Breakfast

▶ Low- and medium-G.I. cold cereal with strawberry milk

▶ Oatmeal with raisins and a drizzle of maple syrup

▶ Orange sections, banana slices

▶ Whole-wheat French toast with Nutella

▶ Vanilla milk with malt powder

Lunch

▶ Sandwiches on whole-grain bread: peanut butter and banana, tuna salad (chopped celery and bread and butter pickles, mayonnaise, lemon juice), chicken or turkey breast

▶ Raw carrot sticks wrapped with thin slices of salami or ham

▶ Fresh fruit: grapes, cherries, clementines

▶ Low- to medium-G.I. cookies

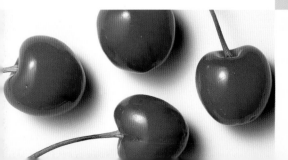

Cooking for kids is easy: Make it colorful, make it interesting, let them eat it with their hands.

Dinner

Pita pizza: Separate pocket pitas into two thin rounds. Set out bowls with tomato sauce, shredded mozzarella, and some or all of the following: half rings of onion and sweet pepper, slices of mushrooms and pitted olives, blanched broccoli florets, thin slices of pepperoni or cooked crumbled sausage meat. Let your children assemble their own personal pizzas. Arrange them on a cookie sheet and bake in the oven on "high" until the cheese is melted and the crust is crisp.

Other dinners your kids might like:

▶ Mini-meatballs and bow-tie pasta
▶ Ravioli with tomato sauce
▶ Chunks of boneless chicken breast grilled on skewers, served with peanut butter sauce
▶ Baked ham with confetti coleslaw (shredded red and green cabbage, grated carrots, tossed in a lemony half-mayonnaise/half-yogurt dressing)

Desserts and Snacks

Do-it-themselves yogurt sundaes are generally a big hit: Put out bowls with vanilla or lemon yogurt, butter cookie crumbs, chocolate chips, crushed berries, fresh cherries, raisins, and so on. Set your children up with plastic, stemmed wineglasses and let them assemble their own concoctions.

Other snacks and desserts your kids might like:

▶ Peanut butter on apple slices
▶ Fresh fruit kabobs with vanilla yogurt dip
▶ Chocolate or vanilla pudding, or both swirled together
▶ Low- to medium-G.I. cookies
▶ Chocolate malted milk

Do your children a favor by helping them acquire a taste for healthy food. They'll thank you one day.

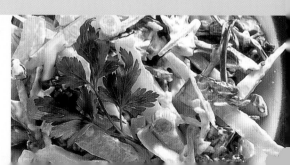

Don't Give Up at Party Time

If restaurant meals are hard, holidays and parties are even harder. It may be necessary to just give yourself a break, with the promise that you'll get back to your best food behavior as soon as it's over. But, as with restaurant meals, it is possible to stay at the low end of the G.I. scale with a little bit of care and planning.

The good news is that half your friends are probably already following carbohydrate-conscious diets and the other half know they should be. That means you will most likely find low- and medium-G.I. choices at most gatherings. If you're in any doubt, mention to your host when you R.S.V.P. to the invitation that you're eating according to the G.I. and discuss the sorts of things you can eat.

Of course, if you're the one actually throwing the party, you can lay out a sumptuous feast that will delight everyone, whether they know about the G.I. or not.

Brunch

Is it possible to eat brunch without bagels? Of course it is. Dense and chewy pumpernickel and rye breads can carry smoked salmon and cream cheese proudly. Serve yogurt cheese spiked with scallions instead of cream cheese, and you'll be way ahead of the game.

Brunchables

▶ Omelet station with chopped smoked salmon, pastrami, sautéed onions and mushrooms, shredded cheese, and sweet and hot peppers

▶ Bread basket with a selection of dense and chewy whole-grain breads and fruity bran muffins

▶ A selection of yogurt, goat or cream cheese spreads thinned with skim milk and blended with fresh herbs and coarsely ground black pepper, chopped smoked salmon, black olive paste, finely diced radishes and carrots, or orange zest and a bit of orange juice, cinnamon and allspice

▶ Fish, smoked and otherwise: salmon, whitefish, sable, herring with chopped sweet onions and caper garnish

▶ Fresh fruit salad: cantaloupe, berries, mango, peaches, plums, with lime juice and grated ginger

▶ Beverages: coffee (plain and flavored), tea (black, green, and herbal), and orange, grapefruit, and tomato juices (with alcoholic beverages, if you wish)

A Dessert Party

Guess what?—many cakes and ice creams are actually low to medium G.I. They may be high in fat and calories, but the damage can be limited if you keep your portion modest.

Sweets can be elegant and delicious even at the low end of the G.I.

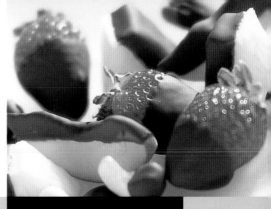

A Children's Birthday Party

Lay out on a plastic tablecloth unfrosted chocolate, vanilla, or marble cupcakes and a selection of tub frostings and toppings like chocolate sprinkles, white and milk chocolate chips, raisins, chopped dried apples and apricots, and crushed mint LifeSavers. Give the children paper plates and plastic knives and spoons. Let them decorate their own cupcakes. The more time they spend playing with their food, the less time they'll have to eat too much. Serve chocolate and strawberry milk to order.

An Adult Dessert Party

▶ Trifle made with sponge cake soaked in orange juice, crushed strawberries, and vanilla pudding

▶ Individual lemon tarts

▶ Ladyfinger eclairs with vanilla or chocolate pudding filling and bittersweet chocolate glaze

▶ Chocolate, vanilla, marble, or banana cakes

▶ Petits fours made with squares of pound cake and bittersweet chocolate glaze with white chocolate detailing

▶ Butter cookies

▶ Chocolate-dipped strawberries and orange sections

▶ A selection of coffees and teas

Cocktail Parties

Whether you are a drinker or not, you may find yourself attending a predinner party involving alcohol and nibbles as a social or business obligation. Cocktail parties can be fun, but they can also be perilous for people trying to control their weight and eating behavior. The relaxing of attention that accompanies a drink or two may lead to overeating. And then there's the added problem that more than a few hors d'oeuvres can quickly add up to an entire meal's worth of food.

Overall, the best defense is to view the opportunity to meet and greet as the main event, while the food and drink are just the side show. Circulate, talk to people, enjoy the gathering, and nurse your drink. If you are drinking alcohol, be sure to get something solid into your stomach early on, perhaps having a small snack before you arrive at your host's house. Pay attention to what and how much you eat at the party, and if it adds up to dinner, don't have another evening main meal afterward. Instead, have a low-G.I. snack later in the evening.

If it's your party, you will have laid out plenty of low-G.I. nibbles and you may be too busy to eat or drink anyway. If you're a guest, you may have to pick and choose. These days, with carb-consciousness on the rise, the chances are that you'll find more than enough to satisfy your appetite without straying out of the G.I. safety zone. Whether you're host or guest, here's a baker's dozen cocktail party ideas just for starters.

G.I.-Safe Hors D'oeuvres

▶ Broiled mushrooms stuffed with baba ghanoush
▶ Caviar on cucumber slices with a dab of crème fraîche
▶ Ceviche in shot glasses
▶ A cheese platter accompanied by dense pumpernickel and rye bread rounds
▶ Deviled eggs with capers
▶ Endive boats with yogurt cheese and chopped spinach filling

▶ Gazpacho in shot glasses
▶ Marinated mushrooms
▶ Mixed nuts
▶ Olives
▶ Raw vegetable platter with fresh herb-yogurt cheese, guacamole, and/or creamy salsa dips
▶ Shrimp
▶ Sushi and sashimi

The gi Handbook

Alcohol, by itself, is a no-G.I. beverage. You can even have a glass of beer without worrying. Sugary mixers will raise the G.I., so it is best to stick with wine and distilled spirits, drunk straight or with soda, seltzer, or tomato juice.

But how does alcohol fit into a health-conscious diet? Most experts agree that a moderate intake of alcohol is acceptable for many people. The key word is *moderate*. That is generally understood to mean not more than one drink for women and two for men each day. As with everything else, pay attention to serving size—if you are drinking giant margaritas, don't fool yourself into thinking that you are having one drink—and make sure you add those calories to your daily intake. Whether you do or not, your body certainly will.

The Bar

Here are some suggestions for stocking your bar:

▶ Mixers and soft drinks: tomato juice, clam juice, orange juice, pineapple juice; seltzer, club soda, a variety of diet sodas, and water

▶ Garnishes: lemon and lime wedges and twists, olives, pickled onions, Tabasco sauce, Worcestershire sauce, and lime juice

▶ Red and white wine, champagne or sparkling wine, and distilled spirits

▶ Ice

For the record, here's what's considered a single serving of alcohol:

▶ 12 ounces of beer

▶ 1½ ounces of distilled spirits

▶ 6 ounces of wine

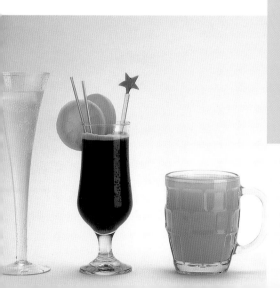

Drink in moderation, if you choose to drink. A glass of wine is fine, so is a beer, but beware of sweet cocktails and sugary mixers. At party time, nurse your drink to make it last.

On the Run

If you are constantly on the move, carry this book and your G.I. awareness with you wherever you go. Many hotels and restaurants now have low-carb choices on their menus in response to diet trends, but the choice is always up to you.

Some Straight Talk about Fast Foods

The growth of fast-food chains directly parallels the obesity epidemic. This is no coincidence. They are a world unto themselves—where portion size is a matter of marketing, and where trans fats, sugar, and refined carbs reign supreme.

Some Basic Equipment

If you are operating from home, pack as much as you can and supplement with low- and medium-G.I. purchases. It's easy if you have the following supplies:

▶ Thermos bottles: Wide mouth for soups and other hot food, regular size for hot and cold beverages and smoothies.

▶ Lidded plastic containers: A variety of sizes, for carrying salads, salad dressings and dips, cut fruit and vegetables, and anything you plan to microwave. Most have a measure embossed on the bottom.

▶ Plastic cutlery: Disposable knives, forks, and spoons.

▶ Blue ice: Keep a few small packs in your freezer. Alternatively, a small bottle of frozen water or ice tea does double duty, keeping your food cool for several hours as it melts to become drinkable.

▶ Insulated bags: Some are small enough to fit into a briefcase, tote, or purse.

If You Really Must

Limit your visits and try these strategies:

▶ Study the nutrient content of every item on the menu: There's a copy somewhere behind the counter, so ask to see it. Better yet, you can find this information online for all the major chains, from their web site or on several independent sites. Check the Useful Web Sites (*see pages 168–169*) or type "fast food" into your search engine and you'll be sure to find them. Reading the lists may be all you need to be convinced to stay away.

▶ For breakfast, order an egg and "whatever" sandwich and discard the bread, biscuit, or croissant.

▶ For lunch and dinner, choose salads (with dressing on the side), plain grilled meat (skinless), or thin-crust pizza.

▶ Don't even consider the fries, thick shakes, or donuts.

Summing Up: The G.I. Way to Healthy Living

▶ Eating low on the G.I. goes hand in hand with portion control.

▶ Calories count. If you overeat even low-G.I. foods, you will gain weight.

▶ The glycemic load of what you eat determines how much glucose hits your bloodstream after a meal.

▶ Gradually trade high-G.I. foods for medium-G.I. and low-G.I. choices until you're in G.I.-safe territory.

▶ Keep a food journal and monitor your progress as you make the transition to G.I.-conscious eating.

▶ Keep fiber high and saturated fats low.

▶ Multiple small meals are better than three large ones.

▶ Breakfast is the most important meal of the day. Don't skip it.

▶ Low-G.I. snacks will help you stay on track throughout the day.

▶ Home cooking is the best way to keep control over what you eat.

▶ Stock your kitchen with low- and medium-G.I. staples and you'll never be at a loss for what to eat.

▶ Hit the road instead of the couch after your evening meal.

▶ Help your kids develop G.I.-smart eating habits by involving them in choosing and cooking foods.

▶ There are low- and medium-G.I. choices galore for parties and holiday gatherings.

▶ Anyone can eat G.I.-safe meals away from home. All it takes is a little careful planning.

▶ Remember, fast-food restaurants, delis, and vending machines are danger zones from the G.I. point of view.

▶ The food lists in Chapter 6 are an excellent starting point, but it's also important to understand the principles of the G.I.

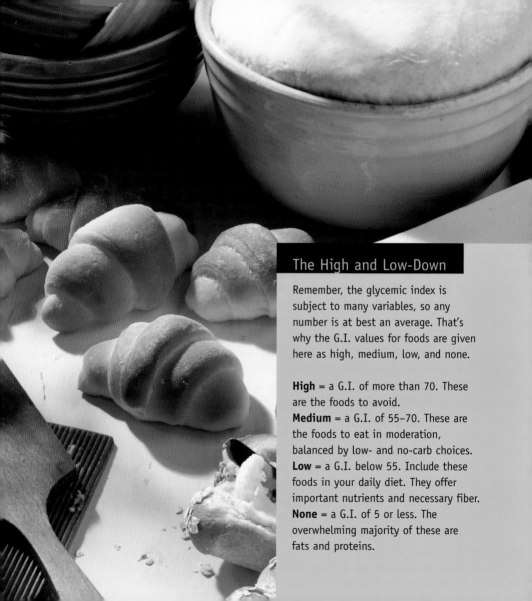

The High and Low-Down

Remember, the glycemic index is subject to many variables, so any number is at best an average. That's why the G.I. values for foods are given here as high, medium, low, and none.

High = a G.I. of more than 70. These are the foods to avoid.
Medium = a G.I. of 55–70. These are the foods to eat in moderation, balanced by low- and no-carb choices.
Low = a G.I. below 55. Include these foods in your daily diet. They offer important nutrients and necessary fiber.
None = a G.I. of 5 or less. The overwhelming majority of these are fats and proteins.

6 G.I. Counts: Rating the Foods You Eat

The lists on the following pages will help you determine the G.I. range of a large selection of everyday foods and ingredients. All G.I. testing is done with a portion of food that contains 50 carbohydrate grams (*see page 28*). That is not the same as the recommended serving size, which may contain a larger or smaller amount of carbohydrate. As always, your best defense against portion distortion is to read the label of any packaged food you eat and then serve yourself accordingly.

What's Included, What's Not, and Why

Unlike caloric values, which are easily determined in a lab, the G.I. is based on complex technology. Fewer than 1,000 foods have been G.I. tested. By contrast, the United States Department of Agriculture's (USDA) Nutrient Database lists more than 8,000 foods. In this book, serving size, total carbohydrates, and total sugar have been taken from the USDA database and/or the manufacturer's label. Fractions have been rounded to the nearest whole number; values of less than 1 are considered to be 0. All values are as precise as possible, but food manufacturers often alter recipes and ingredients. That is why it is vital to read the labels of packaged foods.

The G.I. applies only to carbohydrates, but since this book is meant to help you make wise food choices about what to eat as well as what to avoid, the lists include foods that are primarily fat or protein, or a combination: cheese and other dairy foods, fats and oils, meat, fish, and poultry. Because high-fat foods may represent health risks, anything that contains more than 5 grams of fat per serving is indicated by the 🕑 symbol.

What's the G.I.? Check here before you dig in.

It is impossible to include every single food and ingredient imaginable. Many foods and food combinations have not been G.I. tested; recipes and ingredients vary from brand to brand and country to country; home recipes are not identical to packaged versions. Understanding the principles of the G.I. will guide you when the hard numbers can't be found. Let *carb consciousness* be your watchwords. That way, you won't have to avoid the "good" carbs and all their healthy benefits because you fear they might be the "bad" carbs that flood your bloodstream with sugar.

Guide to Symbols

🔋 High fat (more than 5 grams fat per serving).

❓ If you can't find the food you are looking for, follow the cross-references.

💡 A hint to help you use the G.I. for better eating.

❗ A warning about stealth sugars and other dangers.

🔋 A reminder about G.I. and other nutritional principles.

🏷 Be sure to read the label on packaged foods.

The foods in this section are grouped by type, for easy navigation.

▸ Baked goods (cakes, cookies, donuts, muffins, and pizza)

▸ Beverages (fruit juices, soft and sports drinks, coffee, and tea)

▸ Breads and bread products

▸ Cereals and grains (breakfast foods—including cereals, pancakes, and waffles—and grains)

▸ Crackers, chips, and other snacks

▸ "Diet," "health," and "sports" goods (artificial sweeteners, nutritional support, soy, and sports support products)

▸ Fats and oils

▸ Fish and shellfish

▸ Fruit

▸ Meat

▸ Milk and dairy foods

▸ Nuts and seeds (including nut butters)

▸ Pasta and noodles

▸ Poultry and eggs

▸ Seasonings and condiments (dressings, herbs and spices, and sauces)

▸ Soups, stocks, and broths

▸ Sweets and desserts (candy, ice cream, puddings, sugar, other sweeteners, jams, jellies, spreads)

▸ Vegetables and legumes

The *gi* Handbook

Food	Serving size	Carb total (grams)	Sugar total (grams)	Fat (>5g/ serving)	G.I. rating
Baked Goods					
Cakes					
Angel food	1 oz. slice	17	13		medium
Banana	2¾ oz.	38	27	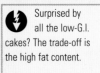	low
Chocolate	3¾ oz.	52	30	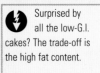	low
Pound	2 oz.	28	17	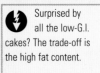	low
Sponge	2¼ oz.	36	17	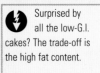	low
Vanilla w/vanilla frosting	2 oz.	58	41	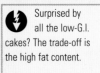	low
Cookies					
Arrowroot	1 oz.	20	4		medium
Butter	1 oz	18	5		low
Graham cracker, plain	1 oz.	22	8		high
Oatmeal	1 oz.	18	5		medium
Petit beurre	1 oz.	22	5		low
Shortbread	1 oz.	19	6	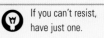	medium
Tea biscuits	1 oz.	22	7		medium
Vanilla wafer	1 oz.	21	8	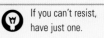	high

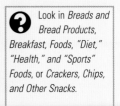 Look in *Breads and Bread Products, Breakfast, Foods, "Diet," "Health," and "Sports" Foods,* or *Crackers, Chips, and Other Snacks.*

Surprised by all the low-G.I. cakes? The trade-off is the high fat content.

How much does a serving weigh? How many cookies = 1 serving?

If you can't resist, have just one.

How much does your muffin weigh? Mega-muffins may count as two or three.

Pizza recipes and ingredients vary, but the trade-off for low G.I. is high fat.

Food	Serving size	Carb total (grams)	Sugar total (grams)	Fat (>5g/serving)	G.I. rating
Donuts					
Cream-filled	3 oz.	25	15	⬤	high
Glazed	2 oz.	27	10	⬤	high
Jelly-filled	3 oz.	33	20	⬤	high
Plain, cake type	1½ oz.	23	8	⬤	high
Sugared	1½ oz.	23	10	⬤	high
Muffins					
Apple-oatmeal	2 oz.	29	10	⬤	low
Blueberry	2 oz.	29	11	⬤	medium
Bran (oat)	2 oz.	24	5		medium
Corn	2 oz.	29	5		high
Pizza					
Cheese	3 oz.	27	0	⬤	medium
Thick crust	3 oz.	24	0	⬤	low
Thin crust	3 oz.	22	0	⬤	low
Vegetarian	3 oz.	25	0	⬤	low
Beverages					
Apple juice, unsweetened	8 oz.	29	27		low
Carrot juice	8 oz.	23	9		low
Chocolate drink, powdered					
• w/water	8 oz.	19	18		low
• w/1.5% milk	8 oz.	32	30		low

Food	Serving size	Carb total (grams)	Sugar total (grams)	Fat (>5g/ serving)	G.I. rating
Coca Cola	8 oz.	27	27		medium
Coffee, black, no sugar	6 oz.	0	0		none
Cranberry juice cocktail	8 oz.	35	35		medium
Gatorade	8 oz.	15	14		high
Grapefruit juice,					
unsweetened	8 oz.	22	17		low
Lemon juice	1 tbsp.	1	0		none
Lemon soda	8 oz.	29	29		medium
Lime juice	1 tbsp.	1	0		none
Malted milk powder					
• w/whole milk	8 oz.	28	23		low
Orange juice,					
unsweetened	8 oz.	26	22		low
Orange soda	8 oz.	32	32		medium
Pineapple juice,					
unsweetened	8 oz.	34	31		low
Strawberry drink, powdered					
• w/water	8 oz.	21	21		medium
• w/1.5% milk	8 oz.	34	33		low
Tea, black, no sugar	6 oz.	0	0		none
Tomato juice	8 oz.	9	7		low

 Look in *Milk and Dairy Foods* or *"Diet," "Health,"* and *"Sports"* Foods.

 You won't find alcoholic beverages in the G.I., but watch out for fruity mixers and sugary garnishes.

 Pay attention to serving size.

 Fruit juice is *not* a source of fiber.

❓ Look in *Baked Goods, Cereals and Grains,* or *Crackers, Chips, and Other Snacks.*

⚡ Whole-grain breads have a lower G.I. than white breads.

❤ Look for dense, thin-sliced breads with visible grains. If it's squooshy, it's not low G.I.

❗ Giant bagels and rolls count as more than one serving.

Food	Serving size	Carb total (grams)	Sugar total (grams)	Fat (>5g/ serving)	G.I. rating
Breads and Bread Products					
Bagel, plain	3½" diam.	38	1		high
Croissant, plain	2 oz.	26	0	❤	medium
English muffin, plain	2 oz.	26	1		high
Flatbread (Middle Eastern)	1 oz.	16	0		high
French (baguette)	1 oz.	15	0		high
• w/butter and jam	2½ oz.	37	0		medium
Hamburger bun	2 oz.	26	4		medium
Italian	1 oz.	15	1		high
Kaiser roll	2 oz.	16	3		high
Pita, plain	6½" diam	33	0		medium
Pumpernickel,					
whole-grain	1 slice	12	1		low
Raisin, cinnamon, nut	1 slice	14	3		medium
Rye kernel	1 slice	12	1		low
Rye					
• cocktail	1 oz.	12	1		medium
• sourdough	1 slice	12	0		medium
• whole-meal	1 slice	14	1		medium
Seven grain	1 slice	14	2		medium
Stuffing (from mix)	½ cup	21	3		high
Taco shells	5" diam.	8	0		medium

The *gi* Handbook

Food	Serving size	Carb total (grams)	Sugar total (grams)	Fat (>5g/ serving)	G.I. rating
Tortilla					
• corn	6½" diam.	12	0		low
• wheat-flour	6½" diam.	15	1		low
Wheat, whole-grain					
• Healthy Choice Hearty	1 slice	18	3		medium
• Hunger Filler					
(Natural Ovens)	1 slice	13	1		medium
• Nutty Natural					
(Natural Ovens)	1 slice	13	1		medium
• 100% whole-grain					
(Natural Ovens)	1 slice	15	1		low
Wheat kernel, cracked	1 slice	20	0		low
White	1 slice	14	1		high
w/1 tbsp. butter	1½ oz.	14	1	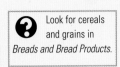	medium

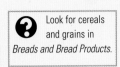
Look for cereals and grains in *Breads and Bread Products*.

Cereals and Grains

Breakfast Cereals

Food	Serving size	Carb total (grams)	Sugar total (grams)	Fat (>5g/ serving)	G.I. rating
All-Bran Original	½ cup	23	6		low
All-Bran Bran Buds	⅓ cup	24	8		medium
All-Bran Extra Fiber	½ cup	20	0		low
Bran flakes	¾ cup	22	5		high
Cheerios	1 cup	20	1		high
Chex					
• corn	1 cup	25	3		high

Food	Serving size	Carb total (grams)	Sugar total (grams)	Fat (>5g/ serving)	G.I. rating
• multi-bran	1 cup	49	5		medium
• rice	1¼ cup	27	2		high
Cocoa Krispies	¾ cup	27	14		high
Coco Pops	1 cup	28	14		high
Corn Chex: *see Chex, corn*					
Cornflakes	1 cup	24	2		high
• sugar-coated	¾ cup	28	12		medium
Corn Pops	1 cup	28	14		high
Cream of Wheat					
• instant	¾ cup	23	0		high
• regular	¾ cup	25	0		medium
Crispix	1 cup	25	3		high
Froot Loops	1 cup	28	15		high
Golden Grahams	¾ cup	25	11		high
Grapenuts	½ cup	47	5		high
Grapenuts flakes	¾ cup	24	5		high
Life	¾ cup	25	6		medium
Oatmeal, cooked, w/water					
• instant	1 cup	26	0		medium
• old-fashioned, rolled	1 cup	27	1		low
• steel cut	1 cup	26	0		low
Puffed rice	1 cup	12	0		high
Puffed wheat	1 cup	11	0		medium
Raisin bran	1 cup	45	19		medium

Food	Serving size	Carb total (grams)	Sugar total (grams)	Fat (>5g/ serving)	G.I. rating
Rice Chex: *see Chex, rice*					
Rice Krispies	1¼ cup	28	3		high
Shredded Wheat					
• regular	2 pieces/1 oz.	38	0		high
• spoon-size	1 cup	41	0		high
Special K	1 cup	22	3		medium
Total	¾ cup	24	5		high
Breakfast Foods					
Pancakes, plain	4" diam.	11	0		medium
Waffles, plain	7" diam.	25	5		high
Grains					
Barley, pearled	¼ cup (dry)	24	0		low
Bran					
• oat	1 tbsp.	5	0		low
• rice	1 oz.	13	0		low
Buckwheat	1 cup	30	0		low
• groats, cooked	1 cup	40	0		low
• kasha, cooked	1 cup	40	0		low
Cornmeal, cooked	1 cup	13	0		medium
Couscous, cooked	1 cup	42	1		medium
Millet, cooked	1 cup	36	0		high
Rice, cooked					
• arborio (risotto)	1 cup	53	0		high
• basmati	1 cup	38	0		medium

 Look for breakfast foods in *Baked Goods* or *Bread and Bread Products*.

Refined grains and flours both score high G.I.

Food	Serving size	Carb total (grams)	Sugar total (grams)	Fat (>5g/ serving)	G.I. rating
• brown	1 cup	33	0		medium
• glutinous (sticky)	1 cup	48	0		high
• japonica	1 cup	38	0		low
• jasmine	1 cup	42	0		high
• white					
• converted	1 cup	36	0		low
• long-grain white	1 cup	36	0		medium
• quick-cook	1 cup	42	0		low
• long-grain and wild	1 cup	37	0		low
• wild	1 cup	32	0		medium
Rye kernels, raw	2 oz.	38	0		low
Semolina: *see Couscous*					
Wheat					
• cracked (bulgur), cooked	1 cup	34	0		low
• whole kernels, uncooked	2 oz.	34	0		low

Food	Serving size	Carb total (grams)	Sugar total (grams)	Fat (>5g/ serving)	G.I. rating
Crackers, Chips, and Other Snacks					
Cheese puffs	1 oz.	15	2	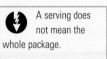	high
Corn chips	1 oz.	15	0	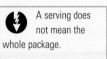	high
Cream crackers	1 oz.	17	0		medium
Crispbread					
• Ryvita	1 oz.	16	0		medium
• Kavli	1 oz.	16	0		high
Melba toast	3 pieces	13	0		high
Popcorn, microwave,					
(plain, unbuttered)	3½ cups	22	0		high
Pop-Tart, double chocolate	1 piece	37	20	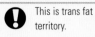	high
Potato chips	1 oz.	15	0		medium
Pretzels	1 oz.	23	0		high
Rice cake, plain	1 piece	7	0		high
Stoned wheat thins	1 oz.	21	0		medium
Water crackers	1 oz.	18	0		medium

 This is trans fat territory.

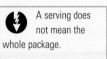 A serving does not mean the whole package.

⚡ "Diet" and "Health" don't necessarily mean low G.I.

🚫 "No sugar added" is not the same as "sugar-free."

❗ Most polyol (sugar alcohol) sweeteners have little or no effect on blood sugar levels, but they may cause digestive distress because of their laxative effects.

Ⓥ You'll recognize a polyol by the "ol" at the end of its name.

🚫 You'll find polyols on ingredient lists, not by themselves as sweeteners.

❗ If you have diabetes, ask your doctor before eating foods containing polyols, especially maltitol.

Food	Serving size	Carb total (grams)	Sugar total (grams)	Fat (>5g/ serving)	G.I. rating
"Diet," "Health," and "Sports" Foods					
Artificial Sweeteners					
Aspartame (NutraSweet, Equal)	1 pkt	0	0		none
Erythritol	10 g.	10	0		none
Lactitol	10 g.	10	0		none
Maltitol	10 g.	10	0		low
Mannitol	10 g.	10	0		none
Saccharin					
(Sugar Twin, Sweet 'n Low)	1 pkt	1	1		none
Sorbitol (Litesse)	10 g.	10	0		low
Stevia	1 pkt	0	0		none
Sucralose					
• (Splenda)	1 pkt	0	0		none
• granular	1 tsp.	0	0		none
Xylitol	10 g.	10	0		low
Nutritional Support Products					
Choice, vanilla	8 oz.	24	9	Ⓥ	low
Enercal Plus	8 oz.	40	11	Ⓥ	medium
Ensure					
• vanilla	8 oz.	40	18	Ⓥ	low
• Plus, vanilla	8 oz.	50	16	Ⓥ	low
• pudding, vanilla	4 oz.	27	20		low
Glucerna, vanilla	8 oz.	29	7	Ⓥ	low

Food	Serving size	Carb total (grams)	Sugar total (grams)	Fat (>5g/serving)	G.I. rating
Soy Products					
Soy milk					
• unsweetened	8 oz.	5	1		none
• w/sugar	8 oz.	8	6		low
• w/maltodextrin	8 oz.	17	13		low
Soy smoothie,					
• unsweetened	8 oz.	7	1		low
• w/fructose	8 oz.	34	30		low
• w/Splenda	8 oz.	7	1		low
Soy yogurt,					
• w/fruit	6 oz.	31	22		low
• plain	8 oz.	22	12		low
Tempeh	3 oz.	14	0		low
Tofu	3 oz.	4	0		none
• frozen dessert	½ cup	20	15	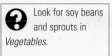	high
Sports Support Products					
Iron Man PR bar	1 piece	25	20	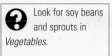	low
L.E.A.N. Fibergy bar	1 piece	23	10		low
L.E.A.N. Nutribar,					
peanut butter crunch	1 piece	20	15		low
Nutrimeal dutch,					
chocolate drink powder	2 scoops	20	12		low
Power Bar	1 piece	45	18		medium
Pure-Protein bars,					
various flavors	1 piece	14	4		low

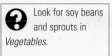 Liven up bland tofu with some low-G.I. herbs, spices, and seasonings.

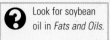 Look for soy beans and sprouts in *Vegetables*.

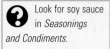 Look for soybean oil in *Fats and Oils*.

Look for soy sauce in *Seasonings and Condiments*.

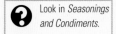

Look in *Seasonings and Condiments*.

"Hydrogenated" or "partially hydrogenated" means trans fats.

Is it saturated or unsaturated fat?

No matter what kind of fat it is, every gram has 9 calories.

Food	Serving size	Carb total (grams)	Sugar total (grams)	Fat (>5g/ serving)	G.I. rating
Pure-Protein shakes					
• various flavors	11 oz.	4	2		low
Fats and Oils					
Baking/cooking spray	½ second	0	0		none
Butter	1 tbsp.	0	0	⊘	none
Canola oil	1 tbsp.	0	0	⊘	none
Chicken fat	1 tbsp.	0	0	⊘	none
Coconut oil	1 tbsp.	0	0	⊘	none
Corn oil	1 tbsp.	0	0	⊘	none
Cottonseed oil	1 tbsp.	0	0	⊘	none
Fish oil, all types	1 tbsp.	0	0	⊘	none
Lard	1 tbsp.	0	0	⊘	none
Nut oil, all types	1 tbsp.	0	0	⊘	none
Olive oil	1 tbsp.	0	0	⊘	none
Palm kernel oil	1 tbsp.	0	0	⊘	none
Palm oil	1 tbsp.	0	0	⊘	none
Peanut oil	1 tbsp.	0	0	⊘	none
Safflower oil	1 tbsp.	0	0	⊘	none
Salt pork fat	1 oz.	0	0	⊘	none
Sesame oil	1 tbsp.	0	0	⊘	none
Soybean oil	1 tbsp.	0	0	⊘	none
Suet	1 oz.	0	0	⊘	none
Sunflower oil	1 tbsp.	0	0	⊘	none
Vegetable oil	1 tbsp.	0	0	⊘	none

The *gi* Handbook

Food	Serving size	Carb total (grams)	Sugar total (grams)	Fat (>5g/ serving)	G.I. rating
Wheat germ oil	1 tbsp.	0	0	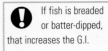	none
Hydrogenated Shortenings					
Crisco	1 tbsp.	0	0	⊕	none
Coconut/palm kernel	1 tbsp.	0	0	⊕	none
Soybean	1 tbsp.	0	0	⊕	none
Soybean/cottonseed	1 tbsp.	0	0	⊕	none
Lard/vegetable oil	1 tbsp.	0	0	⊕	none
Fish and Shellfish					
All fin fish, raw	3½ oz	0	0		none
Caviar	1 tbsp.	0	0		none
Clams, raw	3 oz.	2	0		none
• breaded, fried	3 oz.	9	0	⊕	low
Crab, cooked	3 oz.	0	0		none
• imitation (surimi)	3 oz.	9	0		none
Fish sticks, breaded	3½ oz.	19	0	⊕	low
Lobster, cooked	3 oz.	1	0		none
Oysters, raw	6 pieces	3	0		none
• breaded, fried	6 pieces	10	0	⊕	low
Scallops, raw	3½ oz.	3	0		none
• breaded, fried	3½ oz	10	0	⊕	low
Shrimp, raw	12 pieces	1	0		none
• breaded, fried	3 oz.	10	0	⊕	low
Sushi	2 pieces	37	0		low

 If fish is breaded or batter-dipped, that increases the G.I.

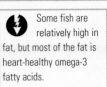 Some fish are relatively high in fat, but most of the fat is heart-healthy omega-3 fatty acids.

Look for fruit juices under *Beverages*.

Fresh and unprocessed is always the best G.I. bet.

Make your own fruit cocktail from fresh low-G.I. fruit.

Gram for gram, dried fruit is absolutely packed with natural sugars.

When choosing canned or preserved fruit, look for the words *water-packed* or *sugar-free*.

Food	Serving size	Carb total (grams)	Sugar total (grams)	Fat (>5g/ serving)	G.I. rating
Fruit					
Apple, raw	1 medium	21	18		low
• dried	2 oz.	26	22		low
Apricot, raw	3 medium	12	9		medium
• canned, light syrup	½ cup	21	19		medium
• dried	8 pieces	17	14		low
Banana	1 medium	27	18		low
Cantaloupe	1 cup, cubed	13	12		medium
Cherries, raw	10 pieces	11	9		low
Dates, dried	6 pieces	40	36		high
Fig, dried	6 pieces	32	24		medium
Fruit cocktail,					
canned, light syrup	½ cup	18	17		medium
Grapefruit, raw	½ medium	10	7		low
Grapes, all types	½ oz.	15	13		low
Kiwi	1 medium	11	8		low
Mango	4 oz.	20	18		low
Orange	1 medium	14	11		low
Papaya	1 cup, cubed	14	8		medium
Peach, raw	1 medium	11	9		low
• canned					
• in juice	½ cup	14	13		low
• in light syrup	½ cup	18	17		low
• in heavy syrup	½ cup	26	24		medium

Food	Serving size	Carb total (grams)	Sugar total (grams)	Fat (>5g/ serving)	G.I. rating
Pear, raw	1 medium	25	17		low
• canned					
• in juice	½ cup	16	12		low
• in reduced-sugar syrup	½ cup	15	14		low
Pineapple, raw	½ cup, cubed	14	13		medium
Plum, fresh, raw	1 medium	9	5		low
Prunes, pitted	1½ oz.	24	12		medium
Raisins	¼ cup	31	29		medium
• golden (sultanas)	¼ cup	32	30		medium
Strawberries, raw	4 oz.	3	1		low
Watermelon	1 cup, cubed	11	9		high
Meat					
Beef, all cuts, cooked	3½ oz.	0	0		none
Lamb, all cuts, cooked	3½ oz.	0	0		none
Organ meats					
• heart	3½ oz.	2	0		none
• kidney	3½ oz.	1	0		none
• liver	3½ oz.	3	0		none
Pork, all cuts					
• fresh, cooked	3½ oz.	0	0		none
• sausage	1 oz.	0	0		none
• bacon	2 pieces	0	0		none
• bits	1 tbsp.	2	0		none
• Canadian-style	2 pieces	1	0		none

 Look for meat fats in *Fats and Oils*.

Unless it is extremely lean and all visible fat is removed, a serving of any kind of meat has more than 5 grams of fat.

Weigh your cooked portions of meat until you are sure what a 3½ oz. serving looks like.

Cured ham and bacon may have added sugar.

Watch out for sugar by any name, as well as for carb-based fillers.

Light, "Lite," and fat-free deli meats may contain more carbs than the regular style.

Food	Serving size	Carb total (grams)	Sugar total (grams)	Fat (>5g/ serving)	G.I. rating
• ham	3½ oz.	1	0		none
Veal, all cuts, cooked	3½ oz.	0	0	●	none
Luncheon and Deli Meats					
Bologna					
• beef	2 oz.	1	1	●	none
• turkey	2 oz.	3	1	●	none
Frankfurter					
• beef	1 piece	1	0	●	none
• beef light	1 piece	2	1	●	none
• chicken	1 piece	3	0	●	none
• turkey	1 piece	0	0	●	none
Kielbasa	3½ oz.	0	0	●	none
Knockwurst	1 piece	2	0	●	none
Liverwurst	2 oz.	1	1	●	none
Pastrami					
• beef	2 oz.	0	0		none
• turkey	2 oz.	1	0		none
Salami	2 oz.	1	0	●	none
Turkey breast	2 oz.	0	0		none
• honey roasted	2 oz.	3	1		none
• smoked	2 oz.	0	0		none
• smoked, fat-free	2 oz.	2	0		none

Food	Serving size	Carb total (grams)	Sugar total (grams)	Fat (>5g/serving)	G.I. rating
Milk and Dairy Foods					
Butter	1 tbsp.	0	0		none
Cheese, all types					
• whole milk	1 oz.	0	0		none
• reduced fat	1 oz.	0	0		none
Cottage cheese					
• nonfat	½ cup	6	6		none
• 1% fat	½ cup	6	5		none
• 4% fat	½ cup	6	5		none
Cream cheese					
• fat-free	2 tbsp.	2	1		none
• regular	2 tbsp.	1	1		none
• whipped	3 tbsp.	1	1		none
Cream					
• half and half	1 tbsp.	1	0		none
• light	1 tbsp.	1	0		none
• heavy	1 tbsp.	1	0		none
• non-dairy creamer	1 tbsp.	2	0		none
Milk					
• buttermilk, low-fat	8 oz.	12	12		none
• chocolate, low-fat					
• w/artificial sweetener	8 oz.	14	13		low
• w/sugar	8 oz.	26	25		low

 Look in *Poultry and Eggs*, *Sweets and Desserts*, or *Beverages*.

 "None" under the G.I. rating doesn't mean "All you can eat."

Look for nut and seed oils in *Fats and Oils*.

Nuts have lots of fiber *and* lots of fat.

Some peanut butters contain sugar and corn syrup.

Food	Serving size	Carb total (grams)	Sugar total (grams)	Fat (>5g/ serving)	G.I. rating
• low-fat (1%)	8 oz.	13	12		low
• reduced fat (2%)	8 oz.	13	12		low
• skim/nonfat	8 oz.	13	12		low
• whole (4%)	8 oz.	12	12	⚡	low
• condensed, sweetened	2 tbsp.	22	22		medium
Ricotta cheese, whole milk	8 oz.	4	2	⚡	none
Yogurt					
• low-fat					
• plain	8 oz.	15	11		low
• fruit, artificial sweetener	8 oz.	15	11		low
• fruit, sugar	8 oz.	48	46		low
• nonfat					
• fruit, artificial sweetener	6 oz.	11	8		low
• soy: *see "Diet," "Health," and "Sports" Foods: Soy products*					

Nuts and Seeds

Nuts

Cashews	1 oz.	9	0	⚡	low
Peanuts	1 oz.	7	0	⚡	low
Macadamia	1 oz.	3	0	⚡	none

Nut and Seed Butters

Peanut butter,					
natural	2 tbsp.	7	0	⚡	none
Almond butter	1 tbsp.	3	0	⚡	none
Cashew butter	2 tbsp.	9	2	⚡	none

Food	Serving size	Carb total (grams)	Sugar total (grams)	Fat (>5g/ serving)	G.I. rating
Sesame seed,					
paste (tahini)	2 tbsp.	4	0	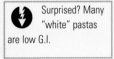	none
Seeds					
Sesame	1 oz.	7	0	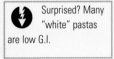	none
Sunflower	1 oz.	6	0	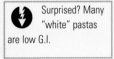	none
Pumpkin seeds	1 oz.	12	0		none
Pasta and Noodles					
Capellini	2 oz.	41	2		low
Fettucine, egg	2 oz.	39	2		low
Gnocchi	5 oz.	45	0		medium
Linguine, al dente	2 oz.	43	2		low
Macaroni,	2 oz.	41	2		low
and cheese, boxed	1 cup, cooked	48	8		medium
Mung bean,					
(cellophane) noodles	2 oz.	40	0		low
Pastina	2 oz.	40	2		low
Ravioli, meat	6½ oz., cooked	38	2	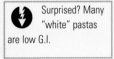	low
Rice noodles (Chinese)	2 oz.	48	0		medium
Spaghetti					
• white, al dente	2 oz.	43	2		low
• white, soft cooked	2 oz.	43	2		medium
• whole-wheat	2 oz.	37	2		low
Soba	2 oz.	41	0		medium
Spirali, al dente	2 oz.	41	2		low

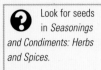 Look for seeds in *Seasonings and Condiments: Herbs and Spices.*

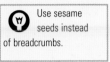 Use sesame seeds instead of breadcrumbs.

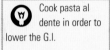 Cook pasta al dente in order to lower the G.I.

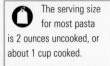 The serving size for most pasta is 2 ounces uncooked, or about 1 cup cooked.

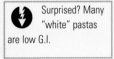 Surprised? Many "white" pastas are low G.I.

Spice up your meals with no-G.I. seasonings.

Many bottled dressings and prepared sauces are made with sugar.

Food	Serving size	Carb total (grams)	Sugar total (grams)	Fat (>5g/ serving)	G.I. rating
Tortellini, cheese	2 oz.	33	1	◉	low
Vermicelli	2 oz.	43	2		low
Poultry and Eggs					
Chicken					
• roasted	3½ oz.	0	0	◉	none
• light meat w/o skin	3½ oz.	0	0		none
• fried	3½ oz.	2	0	◉	none
Duck, roasted	3½ oz.	0	0	◉	none
Eggs	1 large	0	0	◉	none
Goose, roasted	3½ oz.	0	0	◉	none
Turkey, roasted	3½ oz.	0	0	◉	none
Seasonings and Condiments					
Condiments					
Horseradish	1 tbsp.	1	0		none
Hot sauce (Tabasco)	1 tsp.	0	0		none
Mustard	1 tsp.	1	0		none
Soy sauce					
• dark	1 tbsp.	4	3		none
• light	1 tbsp.	1	0		none
Dressings					
Mayonnaise	1 tbsp.	0	0	◉	none
Vinaigrette (homemade)	2 tbsp.	0	0	◉	none

Food	Serving size	Carb total (grams)	Sugar total (grams)	Fat (>5g/ serving)	G.I. rating
Herbs and Spices					
Extracts (vanilla, etc.)	1 tsp.	0	0		none
Ground herbs and spices					
(pepper, nutmeg, etc.)	1 tsp.	1	0		none
Leaf herbs (fresh or dried)	1 tsp.	1	0		none
Powdered spices (cinnamon,					
ginger, turmeric, etc.)	1 tsp.	1	0		none
Salt (plain or seasoned)	1 tsp.	0	0		none
Seeds (caraway, poppy, etc.)	1 tsp.	1	0		none
Whole dried spices (cloves,					
juniper, peppercorns, etc.)	1 tsp.	1	0		none
Sauces					
Pesto	2 oz.	2	0		none
Salsa	2 tbsp.	2	1		none
Tartar	2 tbsp.	4	0		none
Tomato	½ cup	8	6		none
Soups, Stocks, and Broths					
Beef broth/bouillon/consommé	1 cup	1	0		none
Beef stock, homemade	1 cup	1	0		none
Black bean	1 cup	30	2		medium
Chicken broth/bouillon/consommé	1 cup	0	0		none
Chicken stock,					
homemade	1 cup	1	0		none
Clam broth	1 cup	0	0		none

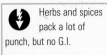

Herbs and spices pack a lot of punch, but no G.I.

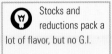

Stocks and reductions pack a lot of flavor, but no G.I.

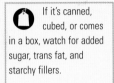

If it's canned, cubed, or comes in a box, watch for added sugar, trans fat, and starchy fillers.

Most desserts are high-G.I. foods, for special occasions only.

Pay attention to serving size and don't go overboard.

Chocolate is low G.I., but packed with sugar and fat.

If you can't say no to sweets, say: "I'll have just a taste."

Food	Serving size	Carb total (grams)	Sugar total (grams)	Fat (>5g/ serving)	G.I. rating
Lentil soup	1 cup	26	1		low
Minestrone soup	1 cup	24	3		low
Split pea soup	1 cup	28	8	●	medium
Tomato soup	1 cup	20	12		low
Vegetable broth	1 cup	1	0		none
Vegetable stock,					
• homemade	1 cup	1	0		none
Sweets and Desserts					
Candy					
Chocolate					
• milk	1½ oz.	26	24	●	low
• white	2 oz.	34	34	●	low
Fruit leather	2 oz.	25	14		high
Jelly beans	10 pieces	28	17		high
Kudos granola bar,					
chocolate-chip	1 piece	20	13	●	medium
LifeSavers, peppermint	3 pieces	5	0		high
M&M peanuts	20 pieces	20	24	●	low
Skittles	30 pieces	29	24		high
Snickers	2 oz.	28	39	●	medium
Twix, caramel	2 oz.	37	27	●	low

Food	Serving size	Carb total (grams)	Sugar total (grams)	Fat (>5g/ serving)	G.I. rating
Ice Cream					
Reduced fat	½ cup	19	17		low
High fat	½ cup	22	21	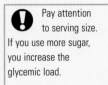	low
Pudding					
Chocolate, instant,					
w/whole milk	½ cup	27	17		low
Custard, from mix,					
w/whole milk	½ cup	23	21	🖤	low
Vanilla, instant,					
w/whole milk	½ cup	28	17		low
Sugar and Other Sweeteners					
Fructose	10 g.	10	10		low
Glucose	10 g.	10	10		high
Honey	1 tbsp.	17	17		medium
Lactose	10 g.	10	10		low
Sucrose (table sugar)	1 tsp.	4	4		medium
Jams, Jellies, and Spreads					
Apricot spread,					
reduced sugar	1 oz.	3	1		medium
Nutella	2 tbsp.	23	20	🖤	low
Orange marmalade	1 tbsp.	14	12		low
Strawberry jam	1 tbsp.	15	14		low

❗ Ice cream is low G.I., but watch the fat, sugar, and calories.

❓ Look for your favorite sugar substitute in *"Diet,"* *"Health,"* and *"Sports" Foods: Artificial Sweeteners.*

❗ Pay attention to serving size. If you use more sugar, you increase the glycemic load.

Look for vegetable juices in *Beverages*.

Shun the starches and find the fiber.

Dried beans are a source of protein and fiber.

Vegetables are a rich source of vitamins.

Most, but not all, root vegetables are high G.I.

If you crave potatoes, then boiled is best.

If you miss mashed potatoes, try mashed turnips, instead.

Food	Serving size	Carb total (grams)	Sugar total (grams)	Fat (>5g/ serving)	G.I. rating
Vegetables and Legumes					
Alfalfa seeds, sprouted: *see Sprouts*					
Arugula	½ cup	0	0		none
Asparagus, cooked	6 pieces	4	1		none
Avocado	6 oz.	12	0	⊘	none
Bamboo shoots, canned	½ cup	2	1		none
Beans, dried: *see Legumes*					
Beans, green, cooked	½ cup	5	1		none
Beans, lima, fresh or frozen	½ cup	17	3		low
Beans, snap, cooked	½ cup	5	1		none
Beet					
• greens, cooked	½ cup	3	0		none
• root, cooked	½ cup	8	7		medium
Bok choy, raw	½ cup	0	0		none
Broccoli					
• cooked	½ cup	4	1		none
• raw	½ cup	2	0		none
Cabbage, green					
• boiled	½ cup	3	1		none
• raw	½ cup	2	1		none
Cabbage, red					
• boiled	½ cup	3	2		none
• raw	½ cup	2	1		none

Food	Serving size	Carb total (grams)	Sugar total (grams)	Fat (>5g/ serving)	G.I. rating
Carrots					
• boiled, sliced	½ cup	8	3		low
• raw	3 oz.	7	5		low
Cauliflower					
• boiled	½ cup	3	1		none
• raw	½ cup	3	0		none
Celeriac (celery root)					
• cooked	½ cup	5	0		none
• raw	½ cup	7	1		none
Celery, raw	1 piece	1	0		none
Chard, swiss, cooked	½ cup	4	2		none
Chicory (escarole), raw	½ cup	2	0		none
Collards, cooked	½ cup	4	0		none
Corn, cooked	½ cup	20	2		medium
Cucumber	½ cup, sliced	1	1		none
Dandelion greens, cooked	½ cup	3	0		none
Edamame: see Soy beans					
Eggplant, raw	½ cup, cubed	2	1		none
Endive, raw	½ cup	1	0		none
Fennel bulb, raw	½ cup	4	0		none
Garbanzo beans: see Legumes: Chickpeas					
Garlic, raw	1 clove	1	0		none
Grape leaves, stuffed	5 pieces	15	2		low
Hearts of palm, canned	1 piece	1	0		none

Food	Serving size	Carb total (grams)	Sugar total (grams)	Fat (>5g/serving)	G.I. rating
Jicama	½ cup	5	1		none
Kale, cooked	½ cup	4	1		none
Legumes (dried, cooked, unless otherwise noted)					
• Baked beans, canned	½ cup	30	10		medium
• Black beans	½ cup	20	0		low
• Black-eye peas	½ cup	18	0		low
• Broad beans	½ cup	16	2		high
• Butter beans	½ cup	16	0		low
• Channa dal (Indian chickpeas)	½ cup	18	0		low
• Chickpeas (garbanzo beans)	½ cup	22	4		low
• hummus	½ cup	25	0		low
• Cowpeas	½ cup	18	0		low
• Haricot beans	½ cup	24	0		low
• Kidney beans	½ cup	20	0		low
• Lentils	½ cup	20	2		low
• Mung beans	½ cup	17	0		low
• sprouts, raw: see Sprouts					
• Navy beans	½ cup	24	0		low
• Peas, split	½ cup	19	3		low
• Pigeon peas	½ cup	20	0		low
• Pinto beans	½ cup	22	0		low
• Romano (white) beans	½ cup	28	0		low
• Soy beans	½ cup	8	0		low
• fresh, boiled (edamame)	½ cup	8	1		low

Food	Serving size	Carb total (grams)	Sugar total (grams)	Fat (>5g/ serving)	G.I. rating
Lettuce, all types	1 cup	1	1		none
Mushrooms, all types					
(except shiitake)	3 oz.	4	1		none
Mustard greens, cooked	½ cup	1	0		none
Nopales (prickly pear					
cactus), cooked	1 cup	5	2		none
Okra					
• breaded, fried	3 oz.	15	5	❤	low
• raw	½ cup	5	1		none
Olives, all types	5 pieces	0	0		none
Onion, raw	½ cup, chopped	7	5		low
• spring onion: *see Scallion*					
Parsnip, cooked	½ cup	13	4		high
Peas, green					
• canned	½ cup	11	4		low
• frozen	½ cup	11	3		low
• raw	½ cup	10	4		low
Peppers, all types	½ cup	3	1		none
Pickles					
• bread and butter	5 pieces	4	3		none
• dill	1 oz.	0	0		none
Potato					
• baked	1 medium	33	2		high
• boiled	5 oz.	28	1		medium
• french fried	5 oz.	60	0	❤	high

Food	Serving size	Carb total (grams)	Sugar total (grams)	Fat (>5g/serving)	G.I. rating
• instant mashed	½ cup	16	0	❤	high
• mashed	½ cup	17	1		high
Pumpkin, cooked	½ cup	6	1		high
Purslane, raw	½ cup	4	0		none
Radicchio, raw	½ cup	1	0		none
Radish, raw	5 pieces	0	0		none
Rhubarb, raw	1 cup	7	0		none
Rutabaga (swede, yellow turnip)	½ cup, cubed	7	5		high
Sauerkraut	½ cup	5	0		none
Scallions, raw	½ cup, chopped	4	2		none
Seaweed					
• kelp/kombu	3½ oz.	10	0		none
• laver/nori	1 sheet	0	0		none
Shallot, raw, chopped	1 tbsp.	2	0		none
Snow peas, raw	½ cup	4	0		none
Spinach, cooked	½ cup	3	0		none
Sprouts					
• alfalfa	½ cup	0	0		none
• lentil	½ cup	5	1		low
• mung bean	½ cup	3	1		low
Squash, cooked					
• yellow, summer	½ cup	4	1		none
Sweet potato, baked	4 oz.	24	10		medium
Tomatillo, raw	½ cup, chopped	4	3		none

Food	Serving size	Carb total (grams)	Sugar total (grams)	Fat (>5g/ serving)	G.I. rating
Tomato, raw, fresh	1 medium	6	3		none
• paste	2 tbsp.	6	3		none
• purée	½ cup	8	2		none
Tomato, sun-dried	1 oz.	15	3		low
Turnip					
• greens, cooked	½ cup	3	0		none
• white, cooked	½ cup, cubed	4	2		none
• yellow: see Rutabaga					
Water chestnuts, canned	½ cup	9	0		low
Watercress, raw	½ cup	0	0		none
Zucchini	½ cup	4	1		none

Glossary

Amino acid: molecular component of proteins. Protein foods are broken down to amino acids for use by the body.

Antioxidant: any substance that inhibits or prevents oxidation, a process of decay that includes spoilage in some foods and is believed to be involved in some diseases.

Beta-carotene: a yellow-red pigment found in many foods and valued for its antioxidant properties; converted to vitamin A by the liver.

Beta cells: insulin-producing cells located in the pancreas; beta cell defects result in diabetes.

Body mass index (B.M.I.): formula used to estimate the proportion of the body that consists of fat. A B.M.I. of 18–24 is considered desirable, 25–29 overweight, and more than 30 obese.

Calorie: unit of heat that measures the amount of energy in food, used by activity, or stored.

Cardiovascular disease (CVD): group of diseases affecting the heart and blood vessels, including angina, atherosclerosis (clogged arteries), congestive heart failure, coronary artery disease, heart attack, and hypertension (high blood pressure).

Diabetes: a group of metabolic disorders in which the body does not produce enough insulin or cannot use it effectively, causing destructively high blood sugar. The two most common disorders are Type 1, an autoimmune disease, and Type 2, associated with obesity and inactivity.

Electrolyte: one of several salts (chlorine, magnesium, potassium, sodium) found in blood and other body fluids; a normal electrolyte balance is required for health; an imbalance may be caused by a wide range of disorders, including diabetes, and may cause a wide range of disturbances, including dehydration and disorders of the heart and nervous system.

Enzyme: one of many complex molecules that act as catalysts in numerous body processes, including digestion and metabolism of carbohydrates, fat, and protein; present in saliva, as well as in the stomach and intestines; no fewer than 16 enzymes are involved in food metabolism.

Fatty acid: molecular component of fat; the main metabolic breakdown product of both dietary and stored fat.

Glucose: simple sugar ($C_6H_{12}O_6$); the breakdown product of carbohydrate metabolism.

Glycemic load (G.L.): measurement combining the speed and degree of blood glucose elevation based on the quantity (grams) and quality (G.I.) of carbohydrate eaten. G.L. = G.I. x carbohydrate grams per serving ÷ 100.

Glycogen: the form in which the body stores glucose.

HDL: high-density lipoprotein; cholesterol that protects against clogged arteries; often referred to as "good" cholesterol.

Hydrogenated, hydrogenation: the manufacturing process that adds hydrogen atoms to solidify unsaturated oils. It is this process that produces trans fats.

Hyperglycemia: abnormally high blood sugar levels.

Hypertension: high blood pressure.

Hypoglycemia: abnormally low blood sugar levels.

Impaired glucose tolerance: prediabetic state of abnormally high blood glucose levels that have not yet reached the diabetes threshold.

Insulin: hormone secreted by beta cells of the pancreas that governs conversion, use, and storage of glucose; insulin defects lead to diabetes.

Insulin exhaustion: the depletion of insulin or reduction in the number or activity of beta cells.

LDL: low-density lipoprotein; cholesterol type that clogs arteries; also known as "bad" cholesterol.

Lipid: another term for fat; often refers to fat stored in the body or present in the blood.

Macronutrient: the main nutritional components of the human diet: fat, protein, and carbohydrate.

Metabolic syndrome—also called *Syndrome X* and *insulin resistance syndrome*: a group of disorders—including central obesity, high triglycerides, low HDL, high blood pressure and abnormal blood sugar levels—that increase the risk of cardiovascular disease, Type 2 diabetes, stroke, and death from one of these conditions.

Micronutrient: vitamins, minerals, and other compounds that the body requires in very small amounts to maintain health and normal function.

Morbid obesity: B.M.I. of 40 or more that also causes health problems.

Phytochemicals: substances found in plants that are thought to have a variety of beneficial effects, including bolstering the immune system, reducing inflammation, and playing a preventive role in cardiovascular disease and some cancers.

Polyol: sugar alcohol added to food as a non-nutritive sweetener.

Postprandial glycemic response: the rise in blood sugar levels that occurs after a meal.

Reference food: also called *index food*; glucose or white bread in a portion containing 50 grams of carbohydrate; the basis for comparing the glycemic response of other carbohydrate foods.

Resistant starch: the type of starch that is not fully digested until it reaches the intestine, which gives it a low G.I. rating.

Trans fat: see *hydrogenated, hydrogenation*; short for trans-fatty acids.

Triglyceride: fat transport molecule. A high level of triglyceride in the blood is associated with clogged arteries and heart disease, and may also be an early sign of diabetes.

Useful Web Sites

The source of all G.I. data is the "International table of glycemic index and glycemic load values: 2002," by Kaye Foster-Powell, Susanna H. A. Holt, and Janette C. Brand-Miller, published in the *American Journal of Clinical Nutrition* (2002; 76: 5–56). A searchable database of the official G.I. values, including G.I. numbers, glycemic load, and carbohydrate content by serving, can be found at: ziag4.mmb.usyd.edu.au/mainV4a.htm.

Other useful web sites for readers interested in diet, nutrition, and health include:

http://www.aafp.org/x16099.xml
The American Academy of Family Physicians' Interactive Nutrition Screening Initiative: Sound nutritional advice tailored to your individual needs and circumstances.

www.americanheart.org
The American Heart Association. Provides information on heart disease and heart health, diabetes, weight control, and more.

www.cfsan.fda.gov/~dms/foodlab.html
"Guidance on How to Understand and Use the Nutrition Facts Panel on Food Labels," from the Food and Drug Administration. Everything you need to know.

www.diabetes.ca
The Canadian Diabetes Association; information and links, in French, English, Chinese, and large-type versions.

www.diabetes.org
The American Diabetes Association. This site gives information, diet and nutrition tips, recipes, and support for people who are at risk for, or who have, diabetes.

www.hc-sc.gc.ca/english/diseases/diabetes.html
Information on diabetes, with an emphasis on prevention, from Health Canada, the Canadian government's department of health; in English and French.

www.hc-sc.gc.ca/english/lifestyles/food_nutr.html
Food and Nutrition portal from Health Canada; viewable in English and French.

www.hc-sc.gc.ca/english/lifestyles/physical_activity.html
Health Canada's portal for information on physical activity and physical fitness for all ages; viewable in English and French.

www.healthfinder.gov
The U.S. Department of Health and Human Service's portal for health-related information will lead you to medical references, resources, and fact sheets geared to different age groups, ethnicities, and needs.

www.hsph.harvard.edu/nutritionsource/
The Nutrition Source brings you solid information about dozens of nutrition, weight, and fitness issues from the Harvard School of Public Health.

www.ific.org/foodinsight/2000/nd/navigatingfi600.cfm
"Navigating for Health: Finding Accurate Information on the Internet." In-depth advice, with valuable links, on how to find safe, reliable, and authoritative information about health issues on the Web. Essential reading for all Internet users.

www.mayohealth.org
Search for answers to your questions about carb-conscious diets, the glycemic index, diabetes, and more, from the health and nutrition experts at the Mayo Clinic.

www.nal.usda.gov/fnic/foodcomp
The USDA's searchable nutrient database, containing the macro- and micronutrient content of any food you can think of.

navigator.tufts.edu
"The Nutrition Navigator: A Rating Guide to Nutrition Websites,"from the Tufts University School of Nutrition Science and Policy—another must-read site.

www.nhlbi.nih.gov/health/public/heart/obesity/lose_wt
The National Heart, Lung, and Blood Institute's Aim for a Healthy Weight site. Full of useful information and tools, including a menu planner, food and activity journal, and weight-control guidance.

www.nhlbi.nih.gov/health/pubs/pub_gen.htm
This site provides downloadable fact sheets and brochures on a wide range of topics, including easy-to-understand information on cholesterol, high blood pressure, obesity and physical activity.

www.nlm.nih.gov/medlineplus
Information on any health and disease topic imaginable, health news, and an online medical dictionary from the National Institutes of Health's National Library of Medicine.

www.nlm.nih.gov/medlineplus/childnutrition.html
Medline's portal for advice, information, and resources about good nutrition for children of all ages.

www.nimh.nih.gov/publicat/eatingdisorders.cfm
Information and links about eating disorders from the National Institute of Mental Health.

www.nnh.org/products/gnfs.htm
Good Nutrition for Seniors from the National Network for Health.

www.nutritiondata.com
A treasure trove containing B.M.I. and calories-burned calculators, nutrition data for major fast-food chains, nutrient-targeted search tools, diet and nutrition news, and more.

nutrition.tufts.edu/pdf/pyramid.pdf
The Food Guide Pyramid for Older Adults: An updated version of the tired old classic geared to the nutritional needs of seniors.

office.microsoft.com/en-us/templates/
A collection of downloadable templates for food journals, fat percentage calculators, nutrition logs, fitness logs, and other records that may be useful for those who want to keep track of what they're eating and how they're doing.

A similar collection of downloadable templates for Mac users can be found at: www.microsoft.com/mac/resources/templates.aspx?pid=templates

www.s2mw.com/heartofdiabetes
The Heart of Diabetes site is sponsored by the American Heart Association. It provides information, tools, and support for people who have, or are at risk for developing, diabetes.

Index

The *gi* Handbook

Acknowledgments

I thank my mother, Catherine Sugarman, for starting me out in life with good eating habits and, at age 87, continuing to be a role model for eating well, exercising regularly, and living a long and healthy life.

Picture Credits

The author and publishers are grateful to the following for permission to reproduce illustrations:
Corbis: pp. 19, 54, 78, 103, 104, 134
Rita Mass/Image Bank/Getty Images: p. 85
Barry Rosenthal/Taxi/Getty Images: p. 75

The *gi* Handbook